The Best Guide for Living with Type 2 Diabetes

This book talks about the nutritional management of type 2 diabetes.

Preface

Those diagnosed with diabetes in the 21st century are the luckiest group because there is a lot of research on diabetes and its implications on the health of an individual, thereby improving the quality of life of those living with diabetes, unlike the early ages.

This book contains information on type 2 diabetes and provides you with the best sources of reliable information on any nutritional advances to help make informed decisions about how to care for yourself when you have type 2 diabetes. This book assumes you don't have any idea about diabetes there; it well explains all terms for better understanding; however, if you already know what diabetes is, then you will have in-depth knowledge while reading this book.

About the Author

Wellington 365 CEO has managed her condition (diabetes) over the past decade and is glad to share his insights about self-managed diabetes to all.

Wellington is an American nutritionist with a piece of in-depth knowledge about nutrition. He has an MPhil in nutrition while helping diabetic patients achieve good and healthy well-being, which is my goal because of my love and passion for nutrition good health.

Reading this book will help you overcome your challenges with diabetes as it contains relevant information about diabetes and answers to hurting questions about type 2 diabetes which will be of importance to the diabetic patient and their guidance.

CONTENTS

"I have high blood sugars, and Type 2 diabetes is not going to kill me. But I just must eat right, exercise, lose weight, and watch what I eat, and I will be fine for the rest of my life.

Frederick Banting.

Introduction

Those being diagnosed with diabetes in the 21st century is the luckiest group because there is a lot of research on going about diabetes and its implications on the health of an individual, thereby improving the quality of life of those living with diabetes, unlike the early ages. The global prevalence of type 2 diabetes is approximately 8% presently, and it is likely to grow substantially in the next few decades. With an alarming rise in incidence in obese children before puberty. Diabetes mellitus has become a major global public health problem. Approximately seven million people are developing diabetes in both developed and developing countries every year, with the most dramatic increases occurring in Type 2 Diabetes (DM2).

If you have had access to this book, the chances are that you have type 2 diabetes or a friend or relative has this condition. Diabetes can be frightening and devastating if you are newly diagnosed; however, learning about your condition and seeking for support is the best way to stay on top of your condition. A key lexicon of diabetes care is good control, meaning keeping your blood glucose or sugar in a normal range or close to normal through low carbs diet, exercise, and medication.

Managing diabetes requires knowledge, dedication, and reframing from certain lifestyle activities and surrounding yourself with good people who care about you and are willing to support you.

This book contains information on type 2 diabetes and directs you to the best sources of reliable information on any nutritional advances; it provides you with enough information so that you can make informed decisions about how to care for yourself when you have type 2 diabetes. This book assumes you don't have any idea about diabetes; therefore, it well explains all terms for better understanding; however if you already know what diabetes is, this book will increase your knowledge with recent and evidence-based practices to reduce blood glucose levels and prevent complications.

The Ancient Greeks were the first to advocate diet and lifestyle management for people with diabetes. Diet and lifestyle intervention were the only treatment options available until the discovery and use of insulin in the 1920s and suphonyl-ureas in the 1940s. Dietary advice is given for optimizing growth while minimizing diabetes-associated complications. Evidence shows that diabetic patients have more than a decade to avoid any complications of the conditions if changes are made through their lifestyle and have a positive attitude towards their health. Diabetes mellitus and its complications are conditions of growing importance from both the clinical and epidemiological standpoint. Diabetes has life-threatening complications affecting several organs and systems, with increased risk for ocular, renal, cardiac, cerebral, nervous, and peripheral vascular disease. Diabetes is a leading cause of premature disability and death in many developed countries and ethnic groups.

CHAPTER ONE

What Is Diabetes Miletus?

Diabetes comes from a Greek word that means a "siphon." Atreus the Cappadocian was a Greek physician during the second century who named the condition diabainein. He described patients who were passing too much water (polyuria) like a siphon. The word became "diabetes" from the English adoption of the Medieval Latin diabetes. In 1675, Thomas Willis added mellitus to the term, although it is commonly referred to simply as diabetes. Mel in Latin means "honey"; the urine and blood of people with diabetes have excess glucose, and glucose is sweet like honey. Diabetes mellitus could literally mean "siphoning off sweet water." In ancient China, people observed that ants would be attracted to some people's urine because it was sweet. The term "Sweet Urine Disease" was coined. 34.2 million Americans are living with diabetes which means 1 out of 10 persons have diabetes while 88 million American adults are prediabetic with approximately 1 in 3 adults (Prevention,2020). Also, 1.4 million Americans are diagnosed with diabetes each year; the number of Americans aged 65 and up remains high at 25.9%, according to the American Diabetes Association. The rising prevalence of diabetes correlates with the rise in overweight and obesity. Although most often diagnosed in people over the age of 40, type 2 diabetes is becoming increasingly common in children, adolescents, and younger adults who are overweight. Type 1 diabetes accounts for 5–10 percent of diabetes cases.

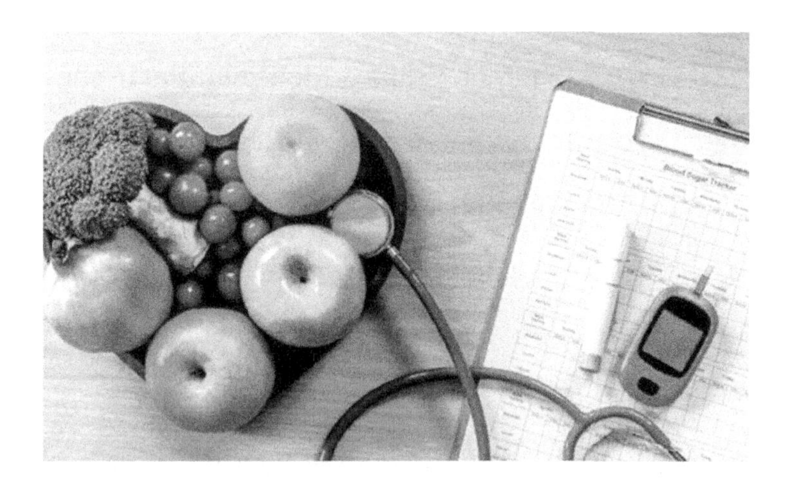

Diabetes, often referred to by doctors as diabetes mellitus, is a group of metabolic diseases characterized by hyperglycemia (increased blood glucose/ sugar level)

resulting from defects in insulin secretion, insulin action, or both. Metabolic syndrome is a cluster of altered conditions that come together in a single person, which increases the individual's risk of coronary heart disease, stroke, and type 2 diabetes. Diabetes can also be defined as a chronic disease associated with abnormally high levels of glucose in the blood (hyperglycemia). The hyperglycemia is due to one of two mechanisms: minimal or no production of the hormone insulin by the pancreas.

After food consumption, the body metabolizes the food substances into glucose. Glucose is a form of sugar in the blood, which is the principal source of fuel for our body. When food is digested, the glucose makes its way into our bloodstream, where our cells use the glucose for energy and growth. However, glucose cannot enter our cells without insulin being present insulin makes it possible for our cells to take in the glucose. Insulin is a hormone that is produced by the pancreas after eating, and the pancreas automatically releases an adequate quantity of insulin to move the glucose present in our blood into the cells; as soon as glucose enters the cells, blood glucose levels drop; however, persons with diabetes have elevated blood glucose (hyperglycemia). This is because the body does not produce enough insulin, produces no insulin, or the insulin is resistant and does not pick up the glucose in the blood resulting in accumulation of glucose in the blood. This excess blood glucose is excreted through urine. Although the blood contains a high amount of glucose, but the cells are not getting it for their essential energy and growth requirements.

Diabetes is said to be a non-communicable and chronic disease because it's mainly not caused by acute infection and mostly results in long-term health consequences, which often create a need for long-term treatment and care; diabetes can only be managed and not cured. Diabetes is associated with obesity because excess body fat that puts an individual at risk of type 2 diabetes as overweight and obesity causes circulating insulin to be resistance to blood glucose as excess fat block the receptors of insulin from binding to glucose in the blood, thereby elevating blood glucose level causing type to diabetes. The long term pre- symptomatic of a marginal elevated and vascular changes in blood glucose levels are known as the prediabetes, which, if not treated can lead to type2 diabetes in 5 to 10years.

Etiology of diabetes

There are several pathogenic processes involved in the development of diabetes, ranging from autoimmune destruction of the pancreas cells with consequent insulin deficiency to abnormalities that result in resistance to insulin action. The anomalies mostly cause diabetes in glucose, lipid, and protein metabolism due to insulin's ineffectiveness on target tissues, Inadequate insulin secretion, and/or decreased tissue responses to insulin caused by insulin deficiency at one or more locations along the complicated hormone action pathways. Insulin secretion and insulin action anomalies frequently coexist in the same patient, making it difficult to determine which aberration is the major cause of hyperglycemia.

The major driving factors of Type 2 diabetes include overweight and obesity, sedentary lifestyle (inactive lifestyle), increased consumption of unhealthy diets containing high levels of red meat and processed meat, refined grains and sugar-sweetened beverages, genetic make-up, and the spotlight is turning to the impact of the intrauterine environment and epigenetics on future risk in adult life. There are clear links among lifestyle, inactivity, aging, obesity, and modernization that contribute to diabetes. There are two forms of risk factors for diabetes which include the modifiable and the non-modifiable risk factors.

Modifiable factors

These are risk factors that can be adjusted for by the individual to prevent type 2 diabetes. People diagnosed with diabetes can adjust their behaviors to manage their diabetes better and lower blood glucose levels, such as changing their diet, increasing exercise, and eliminating unhealthy lifestyle choices (e.g., smoking, drinking too much alcohol, insufficient rest) (Boles et al., 2017).

Unhealthy Diet

This is a diet high in fat and poor in fresh fruits, vegetables, and whole grains are modifiable factors in those who are pre-diabetic, regardless of age. Low-sugar foods may also help to prevent or delay the onset of diabetes. Maintaining normal cholesterol and blood pressure levels may also help to prevent pre-diabetic symptoms and the onset of diabetes. Research suggests that nutritional therapy can help with glycemic management and metabolism.

Recent diabetes research also implies that dietary therapy that is dependent on a patient's insulin level should be evidence-based rather than anecdotal (Franz et al., 2014; Sonestedt et al., 2012).

Nutritional education in diabetes self-management programs is an important part of a diabetic patient's treatment plan.

Overweight, Obesity and Diabetes

Individuals who are overweight or obese are identified by weight and height measurements that produce a body mass index (BMI) higher than normal. Obesity is defined as a BMI of 30 kg/m2 or higher; however, obesity literally means eating more than the body needs, thereby storing excess fats (positive balance), which put one at risk of developing noncommunicable diseases of which diabetes is one of them obesity cause insulin resistance which means there is enough production of insulin in the blood for the transportation of blood glucose into the cell but due to the stress caused by overweight and obesity on the cellular membranes called the endoplasmic reticulum (ER), which in turn causes the endoplasmic reticulum to suppress the signals of insulin receptors, which then leads to insulin resistance and elevated blood glucose levels than to the development of type 2 diabetes.

Lifestyle and diabetes

Certain lifestyle activities such as alcohol intake and smoking and less sleep, and sedentary or inactiveness predispose one to diabetes.

Exercise aids in the maintenance of body weight and blood sugar levels, as well as the reduction of pre-diabetes symptoms. Physical activity has been linked to a variety of health advantages, which are being discovered at a rapid rate. Exercising increases blood circulation, lowers the risk of heart disease and stroke, boosts self-esteem, and lowers whole-body blood glucose levels (Stanford et al., 2015). Because skeletal muscle is crucial for the removal of glucose from the circulation, several activities may help to improve alterations in skeletal muscle. Furthermore, physical activity and exercise have been shown to benefit white adipose tissue (Stanford et al., 2015). Inactiveness has been associated with an increased risk of non -communicable disease due to the excess stores up of fats in the body resulting in insulin resistance and type 2 diabetes.

Non- modifiable risk factors of Diabetes

These are the factors that an individual has no control over, which include sex, age, race, and genetic alterations. Pre-diabetes is more common with the elderly. Diabetes is more likely in those who have inherited DNA alterations in their genome(Boles et al.,2017).

Ethnicity

Pre-diabetes development is influenced by ethnicity. Diabetes is more common in some ethnic groups than others.

Africans, Alaskan Natives, American Indians, Asians, Latinos, and Pacific Islanders are among these ethnic groupings.

Genetics

Both early-onset type 1 and late-onset type 2 diabetes are linked to changes in the DNA. Obese people are more prone to develop prediabetes and diabetes if they have polymorphisms in individual genes in their genome (Karvonen et al., 1993). Polymorphisms in the HLA-DQA1, HLA-DQB1, and HLA-DRB1 genes have been linked to the development of type 1 diabetes in people with diabetes (Karvonen et al., 1993). Polymorphisms in these genes change proteins that play essential functions in type 1 diabetes immune system. Obesity, pre-diabetes, and diabetes are thought to be promoted in human populations by interactions between genetic changes and environmental factors and/or food.

Types of diabetes

The severity of diabetes is determined by blood glucose levels, while the type of diabetes is usually determined by the age of onset. Type 1 diabetes, type 2 diabetes, type 3 diabetes, and gestational diabetes have all been recognized.

Type 1 diabetes

This type of diabetes is also known as juvenile-onset diabetes and insulin-dependent diabetes. It is a progressive autoimmune illness in which the body's own immune system destroys the insulin-producing beta cells in the pancreas. Its onset is relatively swift. Genetic predisposition, as well as environmental circumstances such as a childhood viral infection all influence the onset of type 1 diabetes. It affects 5% of diabetic persons worldwide. After the first six months of life, type 1 diabetes develops. Inherited gene mutations are frequently linked to early-onset type 1 diabetes (Diabetes, 2010). People with type 1 diabetes are dependent on insulin shots to control their blood glucose levels since their bodies cannot produce insulin. To test for type 1 diabetes, it recommended that genetic testing for HNF1A (hepatocyte nuclear factor-1A) will be done to determine T1DM also evidence of non-insulin dependence, such as no ketosis in the absence of insulin treatment or satisfactory glycemic control on modest doses of insulin, indicates a positive result for T1DM.

Type 2 Diabetes

Type 2 diabetes is defined as having blood sugar levels that are greater than normal, which can lead to increased insulin resistance and insulin insufficiency this is when. insulin is present but it cannot do its job of facilitating the transport of glucose into cells. The onset of T2DM is among the older population above 30, and it accounts for 90% of all diabetes worldwide. It mostly influenced by modifiable and non-modifiable risk factors.

The presence of visceral adiposity (excess body fat) is highly linked to insulin resistance. It has diverse effects on muscle, fat, and liver cells. Insulin resistance in fat cells causes the mobilization of stored lipids and an increase in free fatty acids in the circulation. Insulin resistance in muscle cells limits glucose uptake and prevents glucose from being stored as glycogen in the muscle. These metabolic changes cause hyperglycemia. Insulin resistance, which causes high insulin and glucose levels in the blood, is thought to be the cause of the metabolic syndrome and type 2 diabetes, as well as associated consequences. Insulin resistance causes decreased glycogen synthesis and a failure to control glucose production in liver cells, resulting in hypertension.

Symptoms of type 2 diabetes

Frequent urination

When blood sugar levels are high, the kidneys try to remove the excess sugar by filtering it out of the blood. This can lead to a person needing to urinate more frequently, particularly at night.

Increased thirst

The frequent urination that is necessary to remove excess sugar from the blood can result in the body losing additional water. Over time, this can cause dehydration and make a person feel more thirsty than usual.

Frequent hunger

People with T2DM often do not get enough energy from the food they eat. This is because the digestive system breaks food down into a simple sugar called glucose, which the body uses as fuel. In people with diabetes, not enough of this glucose does not move from the bloodstream into the body's cells to be used for energy. As a result, people with

Feeling very tired

Type 2 diabetes can impact a person's energy levels and cause them to feel very tired or fatigued. This tiredness occurs as a result of insufficient sugar moving from the bloodstream into the body's cells.

Blurry vision

An excess of sugar in the blood can damage the tiny blood vessels in the eyes, which can cause blurry vision. This blurry vision can occur in one or both eyes and may come and go. If a person with diabetes goes without treatment, the damage to these blood vessels can become more severe and permanent vision loss may eventually occur.

Slow healing of cuts and wounds

Type 2 diabetes often feel constantly hungry, regardless of how recently they have eaten. High levels of sugar in the blood can damage the body's nerves and blood vessels, which can impair blood circulation. As a result, even small cuts and wounds may take weeks or months to heal. Slow wound healing also increases the risk of infection.

Tingling, numbness, or pain in the hands or feet

High blood sugar levels can affect blood circulation and damage the body's nerves. In people with type 2 diabetes, this can lead to pain or a sensation of tingling or numbness in the hands and feet.

This condition is known as neuropathy, and it can worsen over time and lead to more serious complications if a person does not get treatment for their diabetes.

Patches of dark skin

Patches of dark skin forming on the creases of the neck, armpit, or groin can also signify a higher risk of diabetes.

These patches may feel very soft and velvety, and this is a skin condition is known as acanthosis nigricans.

Itching and yeast infections

Excess sugar in the blood and urine provides food for yeast, which can lead to infection. Yeast infections tend to occur on warm, moist areas of the skin, such as the mouth, genital areas, and armpits. The affected areas are usually itchy, but a person may also experience burning, redness, and soreness.

Type 3 diabetes

Type 3 diabetes has been linked to an increased risk of Alzheimer's disease. Type 3 diabetes is mostly because of cognitive impairment and oxidative stress, which affects glucose metabolism. Its prevalent among people with Alzheimer's disease, such as insulin resistance and mitochondrial dysfunction. T3DM recent investigations indicate an underlying mechanistic linkage between metabolic alterations of carbs, lipids, proteins, and brain dysfunction.

Gestational diabetes occurs when your body can't make enough insulin during your pregnancy. Insulin is a hormone made by your pancreas that acts like a key to let blood sugar into the cells in your body for use as energy.

During pregnancy, your body makes more hormones and goes through other changes, such as weight gain. These changes cause your body's cells to use insulin less effectively, a condition called insulin resistance. Insulin resistance increases your body's need for insulin.

All pregnant women have some insulin resistance during late pregnancy. However, some women have insulin resistance even before they get pregnant. They start pregnancy with an increased need for insulin and are more likely to have gestational diabetes.

Screening Test for diabetes

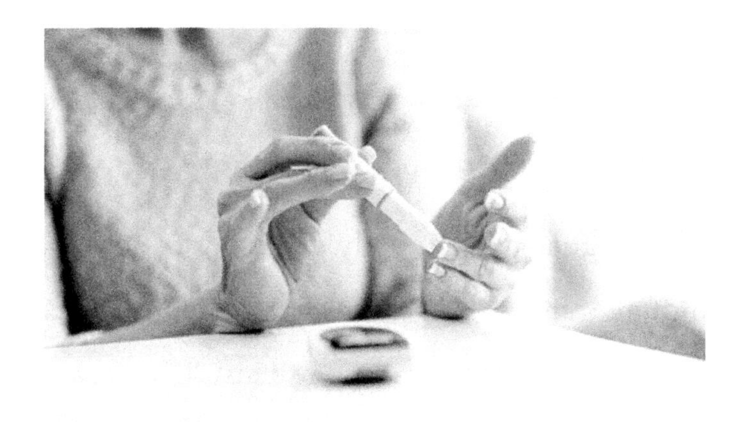

Adults above 45 or earlier should be assessed for type 2 diabetes or prediabetes if they are overweight and have one or more additional risk factors, according to the American

Diabetes Association. Diabetes and prediabetes have several risk factors and for an individual to be diagnosed of diabetes such a person must be tested before, and some of these tests include,

Fasting Plasma Glucose

Fasting plasma glucose (FPG) this test is done eight hours before meals; that's why it is called fasting blood glucose;

therefore (FPG) test should be less than or equal to 5.5mmol/l indicates a normal range.

- FPG less than 5.5 mmol/L is a normal fasting glucose.
- FPG greater than or equal to 6 mmol/L but less than 7.0 mol/L is impaired fasting glucose (indicating prediabetes.
- FPG equal to or greater than 7.0 mmol/L gives a provisional diagnosis of diabetes.

Oral Glucose Tolerance Test

The Oral glucose tolerance test (OGTT) is the gold standard for all glucose tests; however, this test is time-consuming and cumbersome. It is normally performed for patients on the borderline for both the fasting Glucose levels and the random test. This test is carried out overnight the individual ingest 75grams of glucose, and it's assessed between every 2 hours. During an

- OGTT: 5 2-h PG less than 7.8 mmol/L is normal glucose tolerance.

- 5 2-h PG greater than or equal to 7.8 mmol/L but less than 11.1 mmol/L is impaired glucose tolerance, indicating disordered carbohydrate metabolism, leading to diabetes.
- 5 2-h PG equal to or greater than 11.1 mmol/L gives a diagnosis of diabetes

The AIC tests

The A1C test, also known as the hemoglobin A1C or HbA1c test is a quick blood test that determines your average blood sugar levels over the previous three months. It's one of the most popular tests for diagnosing prediabetes and diabetes, as well as the primary tool for you and your healthcare team to manage your diabetes. Because higher A1C levels are connected to diabetes problems, it's critical to meet and maintain your personal A1C goal if you have diabetes.

AIC test result

Normal	Below 5.7%
Prediabetes	5.7% to 6.4%

Diabetes	6.5% or above

Random Blood Sugar Test

This measures your blood sugar at the time you're tested. You can take this test at any time and don't need to fast (not eat) first. A blood sugar level of 200 mg/dL or higher indicates you have diabetes.

Physiological complications of diabetes

Diabetes increases the risk for a variety of major health issues. Untreated diabetes can lead to many health complications, which can be detrimental to an individual's health. What's the good news? Many persons with diabetes can avoid or delay the onset of problems if they receive the proper therapy and make the appropriate lifestyle modifications. Some of these complications include.

Diabetic ketoacidosis (DKA)

Diabetic ketoacidosis (DKA) is a severe illness that can result in diabetic coma (extended periods of unconsciousness) or death. It occurs when your cells don't obtain the glucose they need to function, your body switches to burning fat for energy, resulting in ketones. Ketones are molecules produced by the body when fat is broken down for energy. When the body does not have enough insulin to use glucose, the body's regular source of energy, it does this. The presence of ketones in the blood causes it to become more acidic. They are an indication that your diabetes is getting out of hand. It's mostly caused by Insufficient insulin.

Perhaps you didn't give yourself enough insulin. Or, because of illness, your body may require more insulin than usual.

Inadequate food intake.

When you are unwell, you don't always feel like eating, which might lead to elevated ketone levels. Your blood sugar levels can spike when you don't eat for a while. Insulin response (low blood glucose) If you wake up with elevated ketone levels, you may have had an insulin reaction while sleeping.

- Symptoms of Diabetes Ketosis

- Thirst or a very dry mouth
- Frequent urination
- High blood glucose (blood sugar) levels
- High levels of ketones in the urine
- Fatigue
- Fruity breath
- Lack of attentiveness

Cardiovascular disease (CVD)

Cardiovascular disease (CVD), which affects the heart and blood arteries, is the leading cause of death in individuals with diabetes, accounting for two-thirds of all fatalities in persons with type 2 diabetes. Furthermore, those with diabetes are twice as likely as those without diabetes to develop heart disease or a stroke.

This is one of the diabetic issues you should be aware of; however, there is good news. You can lower your risk of CVD and the issues that come with it by exercising, eating well, and managing your diabetes. Symptoms include.

- Shortness of breath
- Fatigue
- Pain in your; Chest (angina), Throat, Back, Legs, Neck, Jaw, Upper abdomen, Arms, and Weakness or numbness in your arms or legs.

Hypertension (High Blood Pressure)

Blood pressure is the force of blood flow inside your blood vessels. Your doctor records your blood pressure as two numbers, such as 120/80, which you may hear them say as "120 over 80." Both numbers are important. The first number is the pressure as your heart beats and pushes blood through the blood vessels. Healthcare providers call this the "systolic" pressure. The second number is the pressure when the vessels relax between heartbeats. It's called the "diastolic" pressure. Blood pressure is classified into

- Healthy blood pressure: below 120/80
- Early high blood pressure: between 120/80 and 140/90
- High blood pressure: 140/90 or higher

A persistent high blood pressure will increase your risk for heart attack, stroke, eye problems, and kidney disease.

Eye complications

Eye problems and peripheral neuropathy are more common in those with type 1 and type 2 diabetes. You've probably heard that diabetes can cause vision difficulties and perhaps blindness However, most diabetics develop modest vision problems over time.

Glaucoma

Glaucoma is more common in people with diabetes than in people who do not have diabetes. Glaucoma is more likely in people who have had diabetes for a long time. Risk rises with age as well. This occurs when pressure builds up in the eye, glaucoma develops. The blood arteries that the pressure pinches transport blood to the retina and optic nerve. Because the retina and nerve are destroyed, vision eventually deteriorates over time due to the increased blood sugar level.

Cataracts

Cataracts occur in many people who do not have diabetes, but people with diabetes are more likely to acquire this eye condition. People with diabetes are more likely to get cataracts at a younger age and for them to advance more quickly. The clear lens of the eye clouded with cataracts, obstructing vision. Cataracts causes significant vision impairment resulting in lens removal, retinopathy can worsen in persons with diabetes, and glaucoma may develop.

Retinopathy

Diabetic retinopathy is the umbrella term for all retinal problems induced by diabetes. Non-proliferative and proliferative retinopathy are the two main kinds of retinopathy.

Non-proliferative retinopathy (NPR) is a type of retinopathy that occurs when

Capillaries in the rear of the eye balloon and form pouches in non-proliferative retinopathy, the most common type of retinopathy. As more blood vessels get clogged, non-proliferative retinopathy progresses through three phases (mild, moderate, and severe).

Retinopathy with proliferative changes After a few years, retinopathy can evolve to a more serious form termed proliferative retinopathy in certain people. where the blood vessels in the eye is damaged and are closed off resulting in the formation of new blood vessels in the retina. These new vessels are flimsy and prone to leaking blood, which can obstruct vision. Scar tissue might also grow because of the new blood vessels. When scar tissue shrinks, it can distort or pull the retina out of place, resulting in retinal detachment.

Several factors influence whether you get retinopathy

- High blood sugar control
- High blood pressure
- Genes

(Kidney diseases) Neuropathy

Diabetic nerve degeneration can reduce your ability to feel pain, heat, and cold, which can be painful. You may not notice a foot injury if you lose your sense of touch. You could go around with a nail or stone in your shoe all day without realizing it. It's possible that you won't notice if you get a blister. A foot injury may go unnoticed until the skin breaks down and becomes infected.

Changes in the shape of your feet and toes can also be caused by nerve damage. If your foot doesn’t fit comfortably in regular shoes, ask your doctor about special therapeutic shoes or inserts, rather than forcing your feet and toes into shoes that don’t fit and can cause more damage.

Complications of the Foot

Diabetes patients might suffer a variety of foot problems.

Even minor issues might quickly escalate into major concerns.

Nerve damage, often known as neuropathy, is the most common cause of foot problems. This can result in tingling, pain (burning or stinging), or foot weakness. It can also create a loss of sensation in the foot, allowing you to hurt it without realizing it. Changes in the form of your feet or toes, as well as poor blood flow, might cause difficulties.

Poor circulation

Your foot's ability to fight infection and heal can be harmed by poor circulation (blood flow). The blood arteries in the feet and legs constrict and stiffen because of diabetes. Some of the factors that contribute to impaired blood flow are within your control, and smoking causes arteries to stiffen more quickly. Keep your blood pressure and cholesterol under control by following the advice of your diabetes care team.

Warming your feet is a good idea if they're cold. Keep in mind that if you have nerve damage, your feet may be unable to detect heat adequately, making it simple to burn them with hot water, hot water bottles, or heating pads. Warm socks are the best way to keep cold feet warm.

Changes in the skin

Diabetes can create changes in your foot's skin. Your foot may become quite dry at times, and it's possible that the skin will peel and split. Nerve injury inhibits your body's capacity to manage the oil and moisture in your foot, causing this condition.

Calluses

Diabetics' feet get calluses more frequently and at a faster rate. This is due to the high-pressure zones beneath the foot. If you have a lot of callus, you may need therapeutic shoes and inserts. If not cut, calluses can get quite thick, break down, and turn into ulcers (open sores). Attempting to trim calluses or corns on your own can result in sores and infection. Allow a member of your diabetic care team to remove your calluses. Also, do not use chemical agents to remove calluses and corns. These products have the potential to cause skin irritation.

Amputation

Diabetes patients are significantly more likely than non-diabetics to amputate a foot or leg. What is the issue? Peripheral artery disease (PAD) affects many people with diabetes and lowers blood flow to the feet. Furthermore, many people with diabetes suffer from neuropathy, which causes them to lose feeling in their feet. These issues combine to make it easy to develop ulcers and infections, which can lead to amputation. Most amputations can be avoided by checking your feet daily, receiving regular care and visits from your doctor, and wearing proper footwear. Small blood vessels are affected by smoking, and it can reduce blood flow to the feet and slow the healing of wounds.

Oral health and Diabetes

If you have diabetes, you're more likely to develop gingivitis (early-stage gum disease), and periodontitis is deep gum disease and an advanced disease of the gum. Plaque is a soft, sticky substance that forms on your teeth while you eat and primarily comprises germs. Plaque contains around 500 different bacteria, some of which are beneficial to your oral health and others which are not; however, these can be severe and cause an inflammatory response in diabetic patients, especially if you're not meeting your goals, you'll have a higher inflammatory response, which could lead to tooth loss and loss of supporting tissue. The tooth may eventually become so loose that it must be extracted.

CHAPTER 2

Nutritional Therapy Goals And Dietary Management Of Type 2 Diabetes

It's vital to eat well, but it can be difficult to know what to eat and how much to eat, especially if you have diabetes. What we eat and how well we eat can have an impact on our health and well-being. The foods we consume and our nutritional status, including overweight and obesity has been linked with certain health conditions such as high blood pressure, high cholesterol, and diabetes. These illnesses are not only risk factors for NCDs, but they are also major causes of morbidity. Across geographies and societal groupings, nutrition has a critical role in contributing to human health, extending the time spent free of noncommunicable diseases (NCDs), and improving quality of life. Appropriate nutrition is widely recognized as essential for good health and high quality of life. Given the inherent complexity of nutrition, the impact of various dietary interventions, access to high-quality foods, host immunity and infection response, impaired senses (sight, taste, and smell), and mobility are all factors that can limit or increase the body's need for specific micronutrients and influence physiological integrity throughout life as a primary contributor to a long and productive life.

We have achieved significant improvement in terms of lifespan during the previous century through improving healthcare, hygienic conditions, and food variety. Physicians are presumably familiar with Hippocrates' famous phrase, "Let thy food be thy medicine."

Here are some of the goals for nutrition therapy.

- To promote and support healthful eating patterns, emphasizing a variety of nutrient-dense foods in appropriate portion sizes
- To improve overall health
- To improve AIC, Blood Pressure, cholesterol levels.
- Achieve/maintain health body weight.
- Delay/prevent diabetes complications.

- To address individual nutrition needs based on personal and cultural preferences, health literacy and numeracy, access to healthful food choices, willingness, and ability to maintain the pleasure of eating by providing positive messages about food choices only when indicated by scientific evidence.
- To provide the individual with diabetes with practical tools for day-to-day meal planning.

Carbohydrate and Diabetes.

Carbohydrates, sometimes known as "carbs," are getting a lot of attention these days among diabetic patients, and it's no secret that they can alter your blood sugar levels (blood glucose). You might be debating whether you should not eat them at all or even how to eat them. You're not the only one who feels this way. Carbohydrates, protein, and fat are the three main nutrients found in all foods. To stay healthy, you need all three, but each person requires a different amount.

Carbohydrates are broken down to glucose which is the main source of energy for the body, especially for the brain.

Also, they provide the body with other nutrients for good health. All the carbs you consume are converted to glucose. Your blood glucose levels and diabetes management can be affected by the type and amount of food you consume.

However, there are different types of carbohydrates which include those with starch (like bread, rice, pasta, potatoes, yams, plantains, breakfast cereals, and couscous) and those with mostly sugars (like fruits (fructose), some dairy foods (lactose), sweets, chocolate, sugary drinks, and desserts) and the complex carbohydrates or fiber which is mostly in whole grains. Carbohydrates can also be grouped into complex and refined or simple carbohydrates based on their digestibility and their ability to influence your blood sugar levels.

Simple carbohydrates

Simple carbohydrates, such as white flour, sugars, and white rice, are easily digested and release bursts of glucose (energy) into the bloodstream, spiking blood sugar levels. On the other hand, refined carbohydrates have been processed, removing numerous vitamins and fiber. Processed foods are high in refined carbohydrates lacking in vitamins, minerals, and fiber.

Complex carbs take longer to digest and provide a slower, more consistent release of glucose into the bloodstream, lowering blood glucose levels. Some complex carbohydrates include legumes, starchy vegetables, whole-grain, and fiber.

Fiber

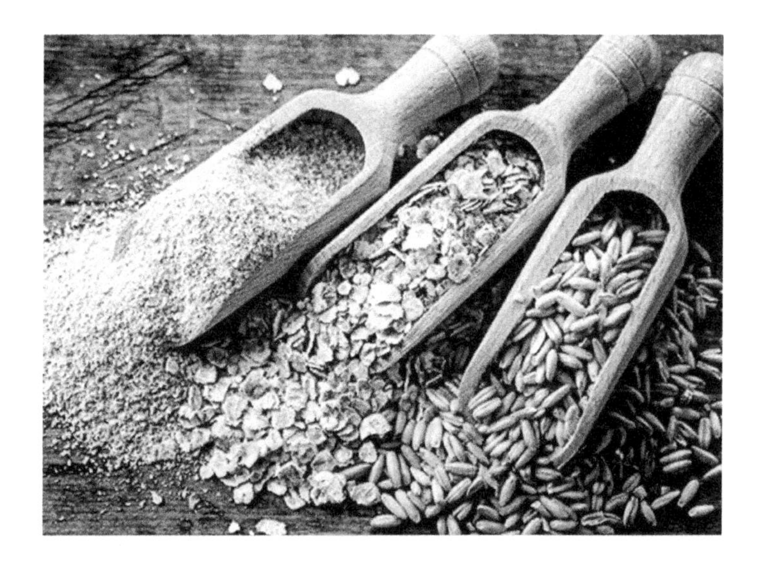

Fiber is a form of carbohydrate that cannot be digested. Whole grain bread, brown rice, wholegrain cereals, fruits and vegetables, nuts and seeds, legumes, potatoes, oats, and barley are all high in these nutrients. Fiber functions as a natural scrub brush for your body, passing through your digestive tract and carrying out a lot of undesirable material with it. Fiber is good for our digestive system, and it can also help keep blood sugar and cholesterol levels in check.

It's crucial to remember that if you haven't been eating a lot of high-fiber meals daily, you should gradually increase your consumption to allow your body to adjust. Gas, bloating, and constipation can result in a sudden increase in fiber-rich diets (particularly those with additional fiber or when utilizing supplements). Make sure you're getting enough water as well because fiber needs water to go through your system.

Sugars

Sugar is another carbohydrate source. There are two major categories:

Sugars found in nature, such as those found in milk or fruit. Added sugars are sugars that are added during the manufacturing process, such as in ordinary soda, candies, and baked products, and these have been associated with health issues such as overweight and obesity, type 2 diabetes or prediabetes, inflammation, and cardiovascular disease when ingested with solid fats results in excess caloric intake.

Sugar Substitutes

There is a plethora of sugar replacements on the market nowadays. The majority of these are non-nutritive sweeteners, which implies that a single serving of the product has very few calories and has no effect on blood glucose levels. These sweeteners can be used in lesser amounts than sugar because they are sweeter. These sweeteners have recognized various sugar replacements as safe for the public, including diabetics. The body does not break down most of these compounds; thus, they pass through our system without providing calories. For some people, these goods are excellent sugar substitutes. A reduction in calories and carbs may result in improved long-term blood sugar, weight, and/or cardiometabolic health.

Carbohydrate and diabetes nutrition therapy

The dietary requirement for carbohydrates is the same for all individuals and diabetic patients; however, the quantity and the type of carbohydrate should be considered.

Since there is no ideal amount of carbohydrates for all people with diabetes, monitoring carbohydrate intake along with blood sugar levels is key to achieving blood glucose control.

- For individuals whose daily insulin is fixed, a consistent pattern of carbohydrates intake with respect to time and amount may be recommended to improve glycemic control and reduce the risk of hypoglycemia.
- Research indicates that low carbohydrate eating plans may result in improved glycemia and can reduce antihyperglycemic medication for individuals with type 2 diabetes; however, this depends on the individual and other medical conditions.
- Emphasize nutrient-dense carbohydrate sources that are high in fiber, including vegetables, fruits, legumes,

whole grains, plantain, starchy roots, tubers, well as dairy products.

- Avoid simple carbohydrates such as sugars, honey, juices, candies, corn syrup, and refined sugars.

Proteins and diabetes

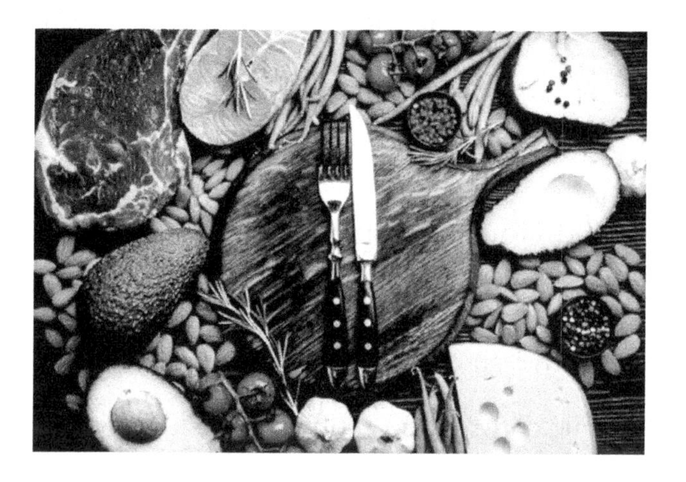

Protein, along with carbohydrates and fat, is one of the three basic energy-producing macronutrients. It aids in the growth of new tissue in the body, which helps to build muscle and repair

injury. Proteins are less efficiently broken down into glucose than carbohydrate, therefore any effects of protein on blood glucose levels occur anywhere from a few hours to several hours after eating you'll need.

Protein is a component of every cell in our bodies and accounts for around a sixth of our total weight. "Protein foods" include fish, chicken, pork, soy products, and cheese, which are all high in protein. "Meats or meat replacements" is another term you could hear.

Diabetic nephropathy (kidney disease) is a condition that affects up to 40% of patients with diabetes. The presence of ketones in the patient's urine is being used to assess kidney impairment in diabetics. Therefore, People with diabetes who have kidney impairment or are at risk of developing it may be recommended to reduce their protein intake.

When eating a predominantly protein-based meal, people with type 1 diabetes or type 2 diabetes on insulin should keep the effects of protein in mind. It's crucial to figure out how your blood sugar reacts to certain foods so you can figure out how much insulin.

Proteins derived from plants

- Quality protein, healthy fats, and fiber are all found in plant-based protein sources. They differ in terms of fat and carbohydrate content, and these include Beans such as black, kidney and pinto
- Bean products like baked beans and refried beans
- Hummus and falafel
- Lentils such as brown, green, or yellow
- Peas such as black-eyed or split peas
- Edamame
- Soy nuts
- Nuts and spreads like almond butter, cashew butter, or peanut butter

Seafood and fish At least twice a week, include fish in your diet.

Albacore tuna, herring, mackerel, rainbow trout, sardines, and salmon are high in omega-3 fatty acids.

Catfish, cod, flounder, haddock, halibut, and tilapia are among the other fish.

Clams, crab, fake shellfish, lobster, scallops, shrimp, and oysters are examples of shellfish.

Poultry

Choose skinless poultry to reduce saturated fat and cholesterol. Cornish fowl, turkey, and chicken Eggs and cheese

In tiny amounts, reduced-fat or standard cheese Cottage cheese is a type of cheese that is made of Whole Eggs.

Beef, pork, veal, and lamb.

It's recommended to avoid red meat, which is high in saturated fat, and processed meats, such as ham, bacon, and hot dogs, which are high in saturated fat and sodium. If you must have these, go for the healthiest options, which are: chuck, rib, rump roast, round, sirloin, cubed, flank, porterhouse, T-bone steak, or tenderloin are all fat-trimmed Select or Choice grades of beef.

Lamb: chop, leg, or roast Veal: loin chop or roast

Pork: Canadian bacon, center loin chop, ham, or tenderloin Excess protein consumption can lead to other health problems although high consumption of red meat has been associated with an increased risk of cancer is more advisable to consume fresh meat in moderation than processed meat, evidence suggests that whey protein consumption of 20g per day will help reduce the risk of type 2 diabetes.

Whey protein and diabetes Whey protein is the byproduct of o cheese processing; it's a rich source of amino acid; however, whey protein is slowly gaining recognition as a functional food and its effect on managing diabetes because of its effect on the guts as the consumption of whey protein aid in slow gastric emptying and stimulate the gut hormones that are important for glucose homeostasis also whey protein can directly stimulate beta-cell from the pancreas to produce insulin, thereby reducing postprandial glycemia (the blood glucose levels after meals). It acts as an appetite suppressor to help in weight management due to its effect on the gut-brain-axis and the hypothalamus(Mignone et al., 2015).

Protein and diabetes nutrition therapy

- Protein consumption for both type 1 & 2 diabetes should at least meet the RDA of 0.8g good quality protein/kg body wt./day as for non-diabetic patient
- At least 1 palm size of protein per meal
- In people with diabetes and diabetic kidney disease is not recommended to reduce the amount of dietary protein below the usual intake; this is because protein reduction can reduce albuminuria but does not alter the course of glomerular filtration rate decline.
- Avoid restricted diets such as ketone diets.

Fats and oils and diabetes

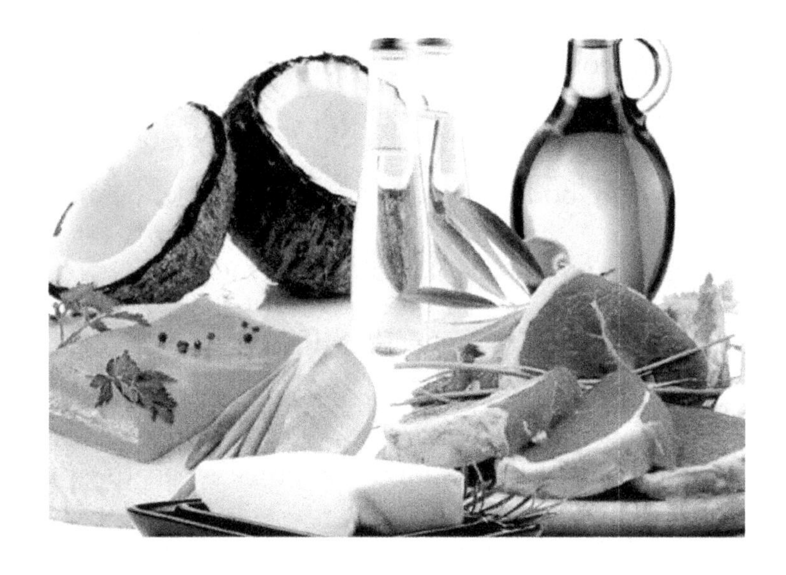

Carbohydrate, sometimes known as carbohydrates, receives the most attention in diabetes treatment. Fat, on the other hand, is an important nutrient to consider as part of a well-balanced diet. Despite what you would think, consuming the appropriate amount of the right kind of fat plays a crucial purpose in our bodies. We all need to eat a nutritious, well-balanced, low-fat diet.

Fat has a significant calorie content, with each gram containing more than twice as many calories as protein or carbs. Eating too much fat might cause you to consume more calories than your body requires, resulting in weight gain, which can wreak havoc on your diabetes management and general health. It's also vital to consider the sort of fat. High levels of 'bad cholesterol' (low-density lipoprotein or LDL) can be caused by eating too much saturated fat, which increases the risk of cardiovascular disease (CVD).

People with diabetes have a higher risk of cardiovascular disease, so making healthy eating choices is even more crucial.

Fat in our bodies serves a variety of purposes, including:

- supplying cells with energy
- producing important fatty acids that your body cannot produce.
- transporting fat-soluble vitamins (A, D, E, and K)
- providing a protective coating around vital organs being required for hormone production

Types of fats

Saturated, trans, monounsaturated, and polyunsaturated fats are the four basic forms of fat. The American Diabetes Association suggests that you consume more monounsaturated and polyunsaturated fats than saturated or trans fats in your diet. A lot has been heard about cholesterol. Most people can't differentiate whether it's good for consumption or not; there are two forms of cholesterol: blood cholesterol is found in our blood, and dietary cholesterol is present in our food. Cholesterol in the blood plays a significant role in the body, as it is the beginning point to produce hormones, cell structures, vitamin D, and other substances. Your body produces cholesterol for these purposes, but it can also absorb a tiny amount from your diet, which only comes from animal sources. Cholesterol found in some foods has a negligible impact on blood cholesterol levels. Food high in dietary cholesterol, such as liver, egg yolk, and shellfish, can be included in the diet, but they must be cooked without fat or with only a small amount of unsaturated fat.

You're more likely to get heart disease if your total cholesterol level is too high. Contrary to popular opinion, dietary cholesterol has a smaller effect on this number than previously thought. Saturated and trans fats play a considerably greater influence in raising blood cholesterol in most people, resulting in an elevated risk of heart disease.

Saturated fats

Saturated fat is an unhealthy type of fat, and this type of fat raises cholesterol levels, increasing your risk of heart disease. One of the fats that we should restrict in our diet is this one. This fat is typically found in animal products and solid-at-room-temperature tropical oils. Saturated fats raise harmful cholesterol (LDL) levels in the body. LDL cholesterol transfers cholesterol from the liver to the cells, and too much LDL cholesterol can cause a build-up of fatty material in the arterial walls, increasing the risk of cardiovascular disease.

Saturated fat is mostly found in animal products such as lard.

- Salt pork with fatback

- Regular ground beef, bologna, hot dogs, sausage, bacon, and spareribs are all high-fat meats.
- Full-fat cheese, cream, ice cream, whole milk, 2 percent milk, and sour cream are examples of high-fat dairy products.
- Butter
- Sauces made with cream
- Using the drippings from the meat.
- Skin of a chicken (example: chicken, turkey, etc.)

Unsaturated fats.

Monounsaturated and polyunsaturated fats are the two forms of unsaturated fats.

They can aid in the maintenance of the body's 'good cholesterol' (high-density lipoprotein or HDL). HDL transports cholesterol away from cells and back to the liver, where it is broken down or excreted as a waste product. Olive oil, rapeseed oil, and avocado have higher levels of monounsaturated fats.

Monounsaturated fat

Monounsaturated fats are considered part of a healthy, balanced diet because of the protective effect they have on our hearts. These fats have been shown to lower our low-density lipoprotein (LDL) cholesterol, an important marker for heart health. Monounsaturated fats are not required to be listed on the Nutrition Facts label.

Polyunsaturated fat

Another crucial fat to incorporate in a properly balanced diet is polyunsaturated fats. This fat decreases LDL cholesterol and your risk of heart disease and stroke in the same way that monounsaturated fat does. Omega-3 and Omega-6 fatty acids are polyunsaturated fats that have been linked to better heart health. Because our bodies are unable to synthesize these fats, they are considered necessary fatty acids and must be provided in a balanced diet. Omega 6 is present in sunflower, safflower, corn, peanut, and soy oils and makes up most of the dietary polyunsaturated fat. Omega 3 oils can be found in oily fish, including mackerel, sardines, trout, and pilchards.

Trans fat

Trans fatty acids have a similar impact to saturated fats in that they raise LDL levels while simultaneously lowering HDL levels.

Milk, cheese, meat, and lamb all contain trace quantities of trans fats. Trans fats are also created when conventional oils are cooked to a high temperature to fry meals, which is why fast food is heavy in trans fats.

The main problem occurs because they are also made by the food production sector using a chemical process called hydrogenation, which converts vegetable oil to solid or semi-solid fats. Artificially created trans fats can be found in large amounts in margarine and partially hydrogenated fat-containing processed foods. It is advisable to consume these processed foods in moderation to prevent obesity.

Ways to limit fats consumption

- Use skimmed or semi-skimmed milk and other low-fat dairy products
- Choose lean cuts of meat and trim any visible fat.

- Remove fat and skin from poultry.
- Swap fatty foods such as butter, ghee, lard, or coconut oils with small amounts of unsaturated fats and oils like rapeseed, sunflower, or olive oils and rapeseed oils spread.
- Choose lower-fat cooking methods, such as grilling, poaching, and steaming or stir-fry with a small amount of oil.
- Limit fatty foods from takeaways

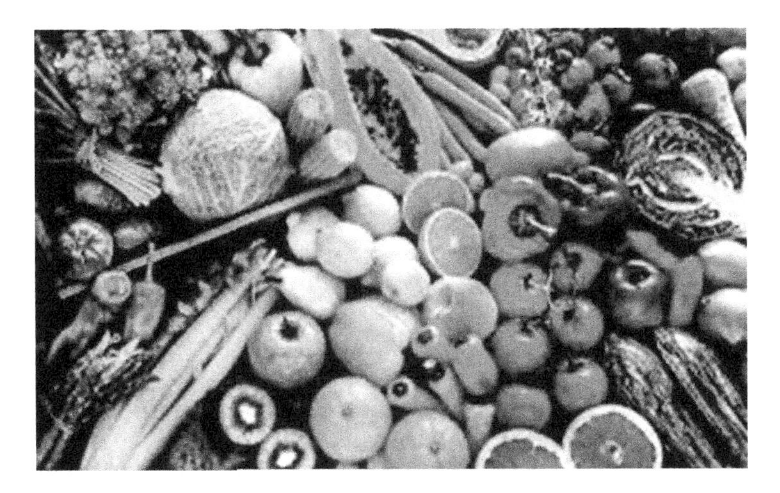

Fruits and diabetes

Fruit and vegetables should be consumed in greater quantities by everyone. You're probably aware of the five-a-day target, which is vital whether you have diabetes or not, and this is because fruits and vegetables are linked to a lower risk of heart disease and some malignancies. Fibre, minerals, and vitamins are also present.

You might believe that fruits are high in sugar content; therefore, it prevents you from eating them. However, the sugar in whole fruit does not count toward free sugars; we do not need to limit this form of sugar. This is not to be confused with the free sugar found in beverages, chocolate, cakes, and cookies, as well as fruit juices and honey. It is very unlikely that you need to reduce your fruit intake, but you could keep a food diary to check how often and how much fruit you are eating. Many people eat fruit infrequently but tend to have larger portions when they do eat them, so some people find that it is easy to overdo the dried fruit, grapes, and tropical fruits. If you consider a serving of dried fruit is only a tablespoon and packs in 20g carbs total sugar, you can see how easily this happens also be mindful of your serving sizes too large banana counts for one and a half portions of fruit and contains about 30g carbs. Therefore, there is the need to cut down on foods with added sugars and refined carbs rather than whole fruit a large banana is still better for your long-term health than a standard slice of cake.

Consume more food! When you have diabetes, you don't typically hear this, but non-starchy veggies are one food type that can help you feel full. Vitamins, minerals, fiber, and phytochemicals abound in vegetables, and with so few calories and carbs, everyone can eat more! Vegetables are divided into two categories: starchy and non-starchy. We're solely going to talk about non-starchy vegetables in this part.

Eat at least three to five servings of vegetables per day for excellent health. This is the very minimum; more is always better!

A vegetable serving is equal to:

- 12 cup vegetables (cooked)
- 1 cup uncooked vegetables

Vitamins and Diabetes

Whether you want to meet your daily vitamin and mineral requirements or treat diabetes complications, there are a plethora of supplements to consider, as well as potential drug interactions, inconsistent information, and safety concerns.

Whether or not a supplement has scientific evidence that it helps with diabetes or related issues, the more important concern is: would take this supplement or vitamin hurt you? Many people believe that supplements have the same vitamins and minerals as entire foods, so why not take a tablet instead? It's because food is the best way to absorb vitamins and minerals.

Consider this: entire foods contain a variety of minerals, enzymes, fiber, and other compounds that may aid in the absorption and utilization of nutrients. A multivitamin is far less healthy than eating a well-balanced meal, and supplements can have a great effect on your blood sugar levels.

Supplements can have unpleasant — or even hazardous — adverse effects, particularly if they mix with your prescriptions. While some components may enhance the effects of your diabetic medications, resulting in hypoglycemia (low blood sugar, also known as blood glucose), others may have the opposite effect, resulting in hyperglycemia (high blood sugar).

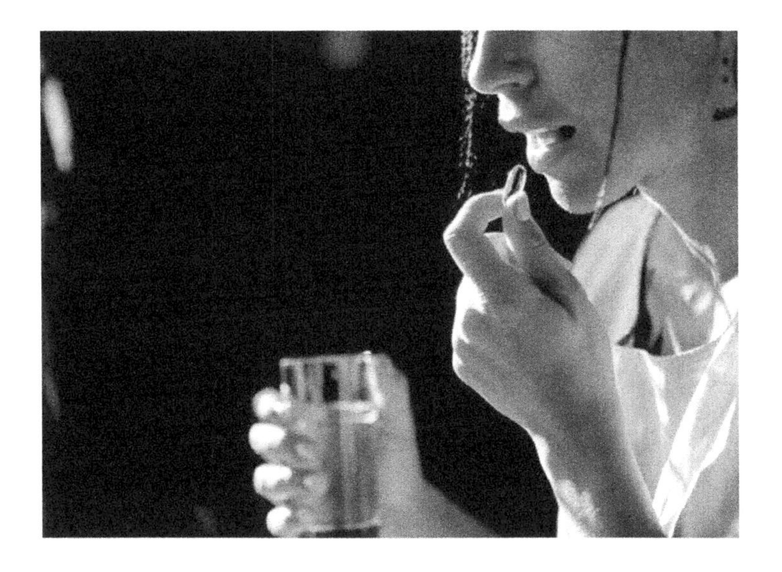

Many supplements have contradictory research. Talk to your doctor before you start taking chromium, vitamin E, St. John's wort, or niacin.

Chromium:

A chromium deficiency can cause high blood sugar levels. If you're deficient in chromium, it's worth a shot, although that's a rare occurrence. If you've been diagnosed with kidney illness, stay away. Supplementing with chromium may exacerbate renal damage and make the condition worse.

Niacin:

Niacin is used to enhance HDL ("good") cholesterol, but it can also have an impact on diabetes treatment. For patients with diabetes, niacin elevates fasting glucose levels (blood sugar levels when you don't eat); therefore, the hazards may outweigh the benefits. While niacin has been shown to increase HDL cholesterol, there is no evidence that it lowers the risk of cardiovascular disease. You can find out if this is safe for you to take by speaking with your health care practitioner.

St. John's Wort with Vitamin E

Vitamin E and the plant St. John's wort can interact dangerously with blood-thinning medicines used to treat heart disease, which puts you at risk of bleeding. Those with heart disease who are taking the blood thinner warfarin have higher amounts of vitamin E in their bodies and are more likely to have bleeding events. St. John's wort has been shown in several research studies to enhance blood thinners' effects. If you're on a blood thinner, stay away from these supplements. These include apixaban, dabigatran, heparin, and rivaroxaban, in addition to warfarin.

Finally, talk to your diabetes team before making any changes, your health care provider may help you figure out if adding a vitamin or supplement to your routine is a good choice.

Dairy and diabetes

Whether you have diabetes or not, we all require dairies such as milk, cheese, and yogurt products or non-dairy substitutes such as soy products daily. These foods are high in protein and vitamins, as well as calcium, which helps to keep your bones and teeth strong. However, some dairy items are heavy in fat and saturated fat, so choose lower-fat alternatives whenever possible or control the portion size.

One portion equal:

- 190ml (1/3 pint) milk
- a small pot of yogurt
- 2 tbsp cottage cheese
- a matchbox-sized portion of cheese (30g)

Adults and older children who consume too much fat may gain weight, and too much-saturated fat can raise cholesterol levels, putting you at risk for cardiovascular disease (CVD). Unfortunately, diabetes raises your risk of cardiovascular disease, so choosing lower-fat products can help you control your risk.

Milk:

It's a smart start to switch to lower-fat milk, such as semi-skimmed milk (green top), from whole milk (blue top), which has the greatest fat. Try 1% fat milk (orange top) or even better-skimmed milk to make a bigger effect (red top). Lower-fat milks have all the benefits of whole milk, including calcium; the only thing you're giving up is the fat.

Cheese :

Cheese can be high in fat and salt, so keep your portion proportions in mind. 30g/1oz – around the size of a matchbox – is the suggested serving size.

Cheddar, Leicester, Gloucester, Lancashire, Brie, Blue cheese, and Edam are all high in fat, with fat between 20 and

40 grams of fat per 100 grams. When reading labels, keep in mind that items with more than 17.5 grams of fat per 100 grams are considered high fat. Cottage cheese, Quark, and reduced-fat cream cheeses are all lower in fat and salt than regular cream cheeses.

Make hard cheese last longer by grating it rather than slicing it, and use mature cheese because it has a richer flavor.

Yogurt and fresh cheese:

Yogurt and fromage frais have a wide range of fat content, so read the label carefully and choose the lower-fat ones. However, that food manufacturers may substitute sugar for fat to compensate for the difference in taste and texture when fat is removed. In addition to the 6—12g of lactose – the natural sugar in milk – a 150g pot of yogurt or fromage frais can sometimes have 20g of added sugar (equal to 5 tsp).

Natural yogurt or low-fat Greek yogurt, which you may sweeten by adding chopped fruit, is a wonderful option for increasing your five-a-day fruit and vegetable diet.

Milk has a lower glycaemic index than lactose (natural sugar in milk), and milk protein slows stomach emptying.

Salt and Diabetes

Even though salt has no effect on blood glucose levels, it is crucial to limit your salt intake as part of your diabetes treatment since too much salt might elevate your blood pressure. High blood pressure is more common in those with diabetes, which raises the risk of heart disease, stroke, and renal disease.

And, if that wasn't enough of a reason to cut back, we now know that eating too much salt raises our risk of stomach cancer. You may simply minimize the amount of salt you eat by being aware of the sources of added salt and following a few simple procedures.

Ways to reduce salt intake

- Instead of shaking the salt cellar over the pan, reduce the amount you use in cooking and measure what you add! As your taste buds adjust to less salt, try to eliminate it entirely.

- Cook from scratch rather than buying manufactured foods and using low-salt foods such as fruit, vegetables, milk, potatoes, grains, and legumes.
- We all have busy lifestyles, so there will be times when we reach for ready meals. Try not to buy them too frequently and read the 'front of pack' label carefully. Choose items with green or amber salt labeling rather than red.
- Don't add salt to the food you've cooked or that you've been served in a restaurant until you've tasted it - this is probably something we've all done – and, even better, flavor your food with herbs and spices rather than salt. We frequently season our food with salt.

Physical activities and Diabetes :

Adults, regardless of whether they have diabetes or not, should engage in at least 150 minutes of moderate-intensity physical exercise every week. At least twice a week, experts recommend doing aerobics, resistance, and strength activities.

Exercise can help to prevent the development of Type 2 diabetes and improve diabetes management. Get active, whether you're at risk for diabetes or just want to keep your blood sugar levels in check.

Before starting a new physical exercise program, consult your doctor if you've been diagnosed with diabetes or any other health issue. If you're on insulin, you'll want to pay attention to your carbohydrate consumption and how you're feeling. Hypoglycemia might occur if your medication dose is not adjusted properly. If you experience low blood sugar, make sure you have a plan and quick-acting carbohydrate supplies on hand.

Increase your training gently, check your blood sugars, and fuel and hydrate before, during, and after exercising, whether you're starting your first fitness program or training for an endurance event like a marathon or triathlon. Your goal is to stay within the blood glucose range that your doctor suggests. You will get higher health benefits as your fitness improves.

Importance of physical activity

- Reduces the likelihood of heart disease
- Regular exercise can help lower blood pressure and enhance high-density lipoprotein (HDL) levels, which can lessen your risk of heart disease.
- Reduces anxiety
- Stress can raise your chances of getting diabetes, and stress can also make it more difficult to control diabetes for people who have it.
- Reduces blood sugar and A1c levels
- When you have diabetes, exercise can help lower blood sugar levels and reduce A1c readings over time. It may also help with protein and lipid metabolism, reducing the risk of organ damage.
- Exercise increases your heart rate
- Being active keeps your heart pounding, which helps your body manage insulin more effectively, whether you're walking quickly, jogging, bicycling, or swimming.
- Improves Blood circulation

Exercise also ensures that blood reaches all organs, including the kidneys, brain, heart, and eyes, all of which can be harmed by poor diabetes control.

Physical activities

Did you know that gardening and dancing are both considered physical activities? Cleaning contributes to your activity minutes as well. Walking (including in the grocery store and mall), stationary and outdoor bicycling, swimming, badminton, mowing the yard, and mopping or scrubbing the floor are all examples of aerobic exercises.

Also, you don't have to complete all your physical activity in one sitting; spread it out throughout the course of the day and week. Start slowly and work your way up from there, then change it up. Remember that you don't have to complete it all at once; start with 5 minutes and work your way up. To keep you going and interested, try a variety of activities.

Resistance exercise is referred to as exercise that improves muscle mass strength, and bodyweight exercises like push-ups and lunges, resistance band or free weight exercises, and everyday activities like grocery shopping and gardening are just a few examples.

Fuel Smart for Activity

To have an effective physical time and result one must also consider their nutrition during their physical activities. Your new fitness routine may necessitate certain dietary adjustments. If you have diabetes, increasing your activity may drop your blood sugar, necessitating a change in your diabetic medication from your doctor. A licensed dietitian nutritionist can also assist you in adjusting your meal plan to ensure that you are getting the proper nutrition for your body. Dehydration can be avoided by drinking fluids before, during, and after strenuous exertion. Drink plenty of water to stay hydrated. During prolonged exercise and in hot conditions, more types of fluids may be required.

Before: A small carbohydrate snack with some protein provides enduring energy for your activity.

During: If you're exercising for more than an hour, you may need additional carbohydrates during activity to prevent low blood sugar.

After: If you plan to exercise for more than an hour, refuel with a post-workout snack.

3-Step Beginner Walking Plan

Step 1: Get Ready!

- Wear comfortable clothes and supportive shoes.
- Set aside time each day for your new activity.
- Plan your route. There are plenty of options to accommodate any weather conditions: an outdoor trail, a gym treadmill, a museum, or a shopping mall. Recruit a friend or listen to your favorite music or podcast.

Step 2: Get Set!

- Go at a comfortable pace for you. Ask your doctor for your safe target heart rate.
- Try setting a goal based on time or distance:

- For time-based goals, increase your time spent walking every two to three weeks until you reach your goal.
- Try adding more distance each day at least three times a week for distance-based goals.

Step 3: Go!

- Keep a record of your daily and weekly time or distance goals and achievements.
- If you have diabetes, also record your blood sugar readings before and after exercising.
- Writing down your progress lets you see your accomplishments and increases your opportunity for success.
- Reward yourself for your accomplishments.

CHAPTER 3

Methods Of Meal Plaining

Meal planning entails more than just deciding what you'll eat. It's all about choosing wise choices that fit your lifestyle and preferences, as well as what's safe for diabetes management.

Once you've mastered the fundamentals, you'll be a pro in no time. It's no easy chore to time meals to keep blood sugar levels in check. There is no such thing as a diabetes diet designed specifically for patients with type 2 diabetes. Diabetes affects everyone differently. As a result, there is no one-size-fits-all diet for those with diabetes.

People with type 2 diabetes used to be sent home with a list of things they couldn't eat after their diagnosis, or they were urged to avoid sugar. However, this advice is to make healthier choices more often and to limit temptations to tiny portions.

Because we know that choosing healthy dietary choices is critical to managing diabetes and lowering your risk of complications such as heart disease and stroke, as well as other health issues such as certain types of malignancies.

Try and make changes to your diet that are reasonable and attainable so that you will stick to them. This will vary from person to person, depending on what you consume currently and what you aim to attain. Consider the following examples of goals, and write them down if it helps:

- To meet my blood sugar target
- To lower my cholesterol (blood fats)
- To maintain a healthy blood pressure
- To maintain a healthy weight
- To be in diabetes remission

With support from your healthcare team, family and friends, or other diabetics, you'll be more likely to meet your goals. There are millions of people with type 2 diabetes who are unsure about what they can eat, and you are not alone. Everyone struggles with lack of time due to the juggling of everything else in life; eating healthy might be difficult. However, planning before shopping, then equipping your kitchen with everything you'll need for a quick meal.

It's critical to make healthier eating choices if you have diabetes and want to lower your risk of complications. We understand that not everyone agrees on which diet is the finest. Therefore, to compile these suggestions, we looked over all the evidence. To make it easier for you to put these tips into practice and to complement whatever diet you choose, we've focused on specific foods.

If you have type 2 diabetes and are overweight, finding a means to lose weight is critical since it improves diabetes control. This is because it can aid in the reduction of blood glucose levels and the danger of other complications. There are several approaches to this, including low-carb, Mediterranean, and very low-calorie diets. Weight loss can help you lower your blood glucose levels, and we now know that significant weight loss can even put type 2 diabetes into remission in some people. You may need to lose, increase, or maintain your current weight if you have type 1 or type 2 diabetes, but it's critical to make healthy eating choices while doing so.

Portion sizes are vital to consider if you have type 1 or type 2 diabetes. It makes calculating nutritional information a lot easier. Keep in mind that serving sizes vary. There is plenty of information to help you if you're feeling overwhelmed by your sentiments regarding food and diabetes. All carbohydrates affect blood glucose levels, and it's critical to understand which foods include carbohydrates. Choose carbohydrate-rich foods that are low in fat and sodium and keep track of your portion amounts.

Here are some carbohydrate sources that are good for you:

Brown rice, buckwheat, and whole oats are examples of whole grains.

Fruits and vegetables, as well as pulses like chickpeas, beans, and lentils, and dairy products such unsweetened yogurt and milk

Similarly, foods low in fiber, such as white bread, white rice, and highly processed cereals, must be avoided. If you're not sure, look at the labels of foods to see if they're high in fiber. This can be done through carbohydrate counting.

Carbohydrate counting

It's critical to keep track of your carb intake if you have type 2 diabetes since you're resistant to insulin and may not create enough of it. It's better to consume a constant amount of carbs at meals throughout the day rather than all at once to minimize blood sugar spikes. Those on oral medicines may utilize a simpler carb counting method than those on insulin.

Carb counting entails counting the number of grams of carbohydrate in a meal and comparing it to your insulin dose at its most basic level. If you use mealtime insulin, you must first account for each carbohydrate gram you consume and then dose mealtime insulin accordingly. To calculate how much insulin you should take to maintain your blood sugar levels after eating, you'll utilize an insulin-to-carb ratio. People on intensive insulin therapy by shots or pumps, such as those with type 1 diabetes and some people with type 2 diabetes, should use this advanced form of carb counting.

While persons with type 2 diabetes who don't take mealtime insulin may not require rigorous carb counting to maintain blood sugar control, some people prefer to do so; therefore, there are a few options, and it really comes down to personal interest, but keep in mind that the ideal carb counting approach for you is the one that considers your medication and lifestyle requirements. A registered dietitian nutritionist (RDN/RD) or CDCES (Certified Diabetes Care and Education Specialist) can assist you in determining what is best for you. If we solely ate carbohydrate items, carb counting would be simple, but most meals have a mixture of carbohydrates, protein, and fat. A high-protein, a high-fat meal can alter how rapidly the body absorbs carbohydrates, affecting blood sugar levels.

Keeping track of your statistics and discussing them with your diabetes care team, which includes an RD/RDN and/or CDCES, is a fantastic approach to understanding how food affects your blood sugar. Continuous glucose monitoring (CGM) or self-monitoring of blood glucose, particularly for insulin dose, can also be beneficial.

How many carbs should I eat?

This is one of the greatest questions asked by most diabetic patients. However, there is no magic number for the appropriate number of carbs in each meal. Your body size and exercise level play a big role in determining how many carbohydrates you need, and hunger and appetite can play a role. Make an appointment with your RD/RDN or CDCES to determine how much carbs you should be eating. They'll devise a diet plan tailored to your needs. Medical nutrition treatment is the name given to this service when a dietitian administers it.

Creating an eating plan may be part of the diabetes self-management education (DSME) sessions. During the lessons, you'll figure out how much carbs you need and how to divide them up between meals and snacks. Everyone's insulin response is different, and we don't want to make the diet anymore restrictive than it needs to be to keep blood sugars under control.

To begin, you'll need to find out how much carbs you're currently consuming at meals and snacks. Tracking your food intake and blood sugar levels before and after meals for a few days will help you and your diabetes care team understand how different meals affect your blood glucose levels so you can figure out the proper quantity of carbs for you.

How do I find the amount of carbohydrates in food?

Reading food labels will tell you how many carbohydrates are in each item. There are applications and other tools available to help you figure out if a product does not have a food label, such as a full piece of fruit or a vegetable. The Food Composition Database of the United States Department of Agriculture, for example, contains nutrition information for thousands of items in a searchable format. The good news is that the more carb counting you do, the better you'll recall the carb level of the items you eat frequently.

When carb counting, you'll want to pay attention to two items on the nutrition facts label:

Severing Size

The serving size relates to the amount of food or drinks that a person consumes on a regular basis and all the information on the label pertains to this precise amount of food. You'll need to account for the extra nutrients if you eat more. For example, if you take two or three servings of something, you'll need to multiply the number of grams of carbs (and all other nutrients) on the label by two or three in your calculations.

Total carbohydrate grams

This figure contains all carbohydrates, including sugar, starch, and fiber. That's right: you don't have to worry about adding on grams of added sugars because they're already factored into the total carbohydrate count! The additional sugars and other bullets below the total carbs list are offered to give you more information about what's in your food. Added sugars, when it comes to counting carbs, you should still aim to minimize the amount of added sugar in the foods you eat.

You should choose foods that are high in nutrients whether you count each carb gram or utilize one of the other meal planning strategies. Vegetables, fruits, whole grains, and lean proteins are examples of whole foods that are unprocessed and in their natural state. Added salt, sugar, carbs, fat, and preservatives are common in processed meals such as packaged cookies, crackers, and other snack foods. While this may appear to be a lot, don't be discouraged; start small and stick to them. Small changes can have a big impact.

One serving = 15 grams carbohydrate

Beans, Peas, and Lentils

Beans, Peas, and Lentils	
Beans, baked	⅓ cup
Beans and peas (cooked) (garbanzo, pinto, kidney, white, split, black-eyed)	½ cup
Lima beans (cooked)	⅔ cup
Lentils (cooked)	½ cup

Milk

1 cup = 8 oz.

Milk	
Chocolate milk	½ cup
Evaporated milk	½ cup
Milk (skim, whole, 1%, 2%, soy)	1 cup
Nonfat dry milk	⅓ cup
Nonfat or low-fat buttermilk	1 cup
Nonfat or low-fat fruit flavored yogurt sweetened with aspartame or nonnutritive sweetener	1 cup
Plain, low-fat or nonfat yogurt	¾ cup

Starchy Vegetables

Starchy Vegetables	
Baked beans	⅓ cup
Corn	½ cup
Corn on the cob, medium 3"	1 (5 oz.)
Mixed vegetables with corn, peas, or pasta	1 cup
Peas, green	½ cup
Potato, baked or boiled	1 small (3 oz.)
Potato, mashed	½ cup
Squash, winter (acorn, butternut)	1 cup
Yam, sweet potato, plain	½ cup

Crackers and Snacks

Crackers and Snacks	
Animal Crackers	8
Crackers, round or saltine	6
Goldfish crackers	½ cup
Graham crackers, 2 ½ inch square	3
Oyster crackers	24
Popcorn (popped)	3 cups
Pretzel twists, mini	15 (¾ oz.)
Sandwich crackers	3
Snack chips (tortilla, potato)	15-20 (1 oz.)

Vegetables

½ cup cooked or 1 cup raw = 5 grams carb

1 ½ cups cooked or 3 cups raw = 15 grams of carb

Artichoke	Leeks
Asparagus	Mixed vegetables (without corn, peas, or pasta)
Beans (green, wax, Italian)	Mushrooms
Bean sprouts	Okra
Beets	Onions
Broccoli	Pea pods
Brussels sprouts	Peppers
Cabbage	Radishes
Carrots	Salad greens
Cauliflower	Sauerkraut
Celery	Spinach
Cucumber	Summer squash
Eggplant	Tomato (canned, sauce, juice)
Green onions or scallions	Turnips
Greens (collard, kale, mustard, turnip)	Water chestnuts
Kohlrabi	Watercress
	Zucchini

Glycemic index and diabetes

The glycemic index (GI) measures how quickly, moderately, or slowly a diet affects blood glucose levels. This means it could be helpful in managing your diabetes. Carbohydrates digest and absorb at different rates, and the GI is a measurement of how rapidly carbohydrate-based foods and drinks raise blood glucose levels after consumption. The GI index ranges from 0 to 100, and the most common reference is pure glucose, which has a GI of roughly 100. Most fruits and vegetables, unsweetened milk, nuts, legumes, some wholegrain cereals, and bread have a low GI value (55 or below). Studies have demonstrated low-GI foods to help persons with Type 2 diabetes maintain their long-term blood glucose (HbA1c) levels.

Low-GI meals aren't always healthy; most chocolates, for example, have a low GI due to their fat content, which inhibits carbohydrate absorption. The overall GI of a meal is changed when items with different GIs are combined. Switching to a low GI option with each meal or snack can help you get the most out of GI. If you're trying to lose weight, avoid lower GI foods like chocolate, which are heavy in calories save them for special occasions. It's not just about GI ratings when it comes to eating for diabetic management. As part of a long-term healthy diet, consider foods high in fiber and whole grains, as well as low in saturated fat, salt, and sugar. diabetes.

If you simply consider the GI of foods and ignore other factors, your diet may be unbalanced and heavy in fat and calories, resulting in weight gain (making blood glucose regulation more difficult) and an increased risk of heart disease. It's crucial to consider the nutritional balance of your meals, which should be low in saturated fat, salt, and sugar and high in fruits and vegetables, whole grains, legumes, nuts, and fatty salmon. The amount of carbohydrates you consume has a greater impact on your blood glucose levels than the GI alone. For example, pasta has a lower GI than watermelon, but pasta has more carbs, so if you eat the same amount of pasta and watermelon, and the pasta will have a greater influence on your blood glucose levels afterward.

The most important thing to remember is to keep track of your portion sizes.

Other factors that influence Glycemic index

- Methods of preparation include frying, boiling, and baking.
- Fruit and vegetable processing, as well as the maturity of specific veggies
- Whole grains and high-fiber diets function as a physical barrier to carbohydrate absorption, slowing it down. This is not to be confused with 'wholemeal,' which contains the entire grain but has been pulverized rather being left whole. Some wholegrain mixed-grain pieces of bread, for example, have a lower GI than wholemeal or white bread.
- A food's GI is reduced by fat. Chocolate, for example, has a low GI due to the fat content, and crisps have a lower GI than potatoes cooked without fat.
- Foods with more protein have a lower GI. Because milk and other dairy products are high in protein and fat, they have a low GI.

Glycemic Index and Glycemic Load of Popular Foods

Green = Low ~ Orange = Medium ~ Red = High

Types of Food	Glycemic Index	Serving Size	Net Carbs	Glycemic Load
Peanuts	14	4 oz (113g)	15	2
Bean sprouts	25	1 cup (104g)	4	1
Grapefruit	25	1/2 large (166g)	11	3
Pizza	30	2 slices (260g)	42	13
Lowfat yogurt	33	1 cup (245g)	47	16
Apples	38	1 medium (138g)	16	6
Spaghetti	42	1 cup (140g)	38	16
Carrots	47	1 large (72g)	5	2
Oranges	48	1 medium (131g)	12	6
Bananas	52	1 large (136g)	27	14
Potato chips	54	4 oz (114g)	55	30
Snickers Bar	55	1 bar (113g)	64	35
Brown rice	55	1 cup (195g)	42	23
Honey	55	1 tbsp (21g)	17	9
Oatmeal	58	1 cup (234g)	21	12
Ice cream	61	1 cup (72g)	16	10
Macaroni and cheese	64	1 serving (166g)	47	30
Raisins	64	1 small box (43g)	32	20
White rice	64	1 cup (186g)	52	33
Sugar (sucrose)	68	1 tbsp (12g)	12	8
White bread	70	1 slice (30g)	14	10
Watermelon	72	1 cup (154g)	11	8
Popcorn	72	2 cups (16g)	10	7
Baked potato	85	1 medium (173g)	33	28
Glucose	100	(50g)	50	50

Nutritional values in this table is courtesy of:
http://nutritiondata.self.com/topics/glycemic-index#ixzz2Jwaw2XZx

Glycemic index cart

Food exchange and diabetes

The term "exchange" refers to food items on each list that can be swapped out for any other item on the same list within each food list; one exchange is roughly equivalent to another in terms of carbohydrate, calories, protein, and fat. A diabetic exchange diet is a list of food serving sizes that you can eat daily, and these foods are categorized into six categories. To keep your diabetes under control, you must consume the recommended number of servings from each food group each day.

Food carbs are converted to blood sugar (glucose) in the body. The body does not produce enough insulin, or the insulin it does produce does not act correctly in diabetes. This results in an abnormally high blood sugar level. Limiting carbohydrates and total calories in your diet can help you control your blood sugar. Maintaining a regular blood sugar level can help you avoid problems with your kidneys, eyes, nerves, or heart.

A diabetic exchange diet is meant to give you easy control over how much sugar and cholesterol you consume. A successful diabetic exchange diet will aid in weight loss, BMI (Body Mass Index), and blood sugar control. Food must be precisely measured in a diabetic exchange diet, and three meals and one snack per day are generally suggested. The diabetic exchange categorizes foods into six categories and weighs them per serving size.

Your nutritionist will create a food plan for you. This meal plan specifies how many servings of each food type should be consumed. And when is the best time to eat them during the day?

During this diet, you will need to weigh your food. Most people on a diabetic exchange diet need to eat three meals and one to three snacks each day. Foods from the same food group can be swapped or traded for one another. For example, 3/4 cup dry cereal can be substituted for 1 slice of bread. Alternatively, 1/2 cup fruit juice can be used for 1/2 of a 9-inch banana.

- The diabetic exchange system is adaptable, allowing you to choose foods based on your calorie needs.
- Calculate your BMI to determine your calorie intake and how many servings of each food type you can consume each day (Body Mass Index).
- If your BMI is normal, you should be able to consume between 1,800 and 2,000 calories each day. This is lowered to around 1,600 for those with an overweight BMI and between 1,200 and 1,400 for those with an obese BMI.
- Upon working out your BMI and calorie allowances, you should then assess how many carbohydrates you can have in your daily diet.
- This can be done by multiplying your daily calorie intake by .43 and then dividing that number by four.
- Exchange = ([Daily Calorie Intake] * .43)/4.
- An example of this would be 1600 x .43 = 688 / 4 = 172 grams of carbohydrate, which would be your daily allowance.

Diabetic exchange list does include a large range of foods to adhere to them; however, some foods that are perfectly safe to eat but may not be included. Diabetic exchange diet patients should avoid foods on the 'Prohibited List; however, just because an item isn't on the restricted list doesn't mean it's safe to eat.

Nutritional labels

Understanding how to read the Nutrition Facts label on food might help you make better decisions. The nutrition label breaks down the calories, carbohydrates, fat, fiber, protein, and vitamins in each serving of the item, making it easy to compare the nutrition of similar goods. Make sure to compare nutrition information from different brands of the same food's nutrition information can vary greatly. For example, for the same serving size, one brand of tomato sauce may have more calories and sugar than another.

Eat more meals high in vitamins, minerals (such as calcium and iron), and fiber in general. Avoid trans-fat and eat fewer meals that are heavy in added sugars, saturated icon, and sodium (salt). Remember that the percent Daily Value of each nutrient, such as the 10% total fat in the example below, is based on consuming 2,000 calories per day. You have the option to choose how much they contribute to what a typical adult requires for each day; however, also consider the gender, activity level, current weight, and whether you're trying to lose or maintain your weight.

Understanding food labels

The traffic light system for 'front of pack' labeling has been available for a while and is a quick method to see how nutritious a meal is. The labels indicate the number of calories in the meal or drink, as well as whether it is low (green), medium (amber), or high (red) in fat, saturated fat, sugar, and salt. The information on the front of the package also indicates how much of the product contributes to an adult's Reference Intake (RI). Choose foods that have more greens and ambers than reds. If traffic lights aren't available, look at the 'per 100g' column on the nutritional label on the back of the package. This 'front of pack' labeling is intended to assist people rapidly determining which foods are healthier based on fat, sugar, and salt content. According to EU guidelines for low, medium, and high concentrations, these nutrients are color-coded. Carbohydrates aren't listed on the front of the package since there are no defined guidelines for establishing how much low, medium, or high carb is in a certain item.

The back of a pack must have information about the ingredients, nutritional composition, known allergens, 'best before' or 'use-by' dates, and the product's weight. The ingredients are given in order of amount, beginning with the highest-quantity ingredient and ending with the lowest-quantity ingredient. If sugar appears at the top of the list, the food is most likely high in sugar. It's also provided other information on nutrients, and these are given in per 100g so that customers can compare two identical products easily. Many goods also include nutrient content per portion information in addition to the per 100g information, which might be valuable for consumers who want to know how much carb they're consuming.

Portion size

Begin by examining the serving size. The serving size is the basis for all the information on the label. If you eat more, you'll consume more calories, carbs, and other nutrients than what's listed; however, the manufacturer's definition of a portion or serving size differs from yours. The serving sizes are generally appropriate for individuals over the age of 18, and different dosages may be required for younger children and teenagers. Even if you make better choices, eating huge amounts may result in you absorbing more calories, fats, and sweets than you require. Your nutrient and calorie intake are influenced by how much you eat of any product, so think about portion size while you're shopping and don't always eat the quantity the manufacturer suggests if you think you need less. Portion size and serving size aren't always the same. A portion is the amount of food you choose to eat at one time, while a serving is a specific amount of food, such as one slice of bread or 8 ounces (1 cup) of milk.

Restaurant portions are now far greater than they were a few years ago, and one entrée might serve three or four people. Studies show that people tend to eat more when they're served more food, so getting portions under control is important for managing weight and blood sugar.

If you're eating out, pack half of your meal to take home so you may consume it later. Measure out snacks at home; don't consume them directly from the bag or box. Keep the serving bowls out of reach at dinnertime to avoid the temptation to go back for seconds. Here is some "useful" guidance, you will always be able to estimate portion sizes:

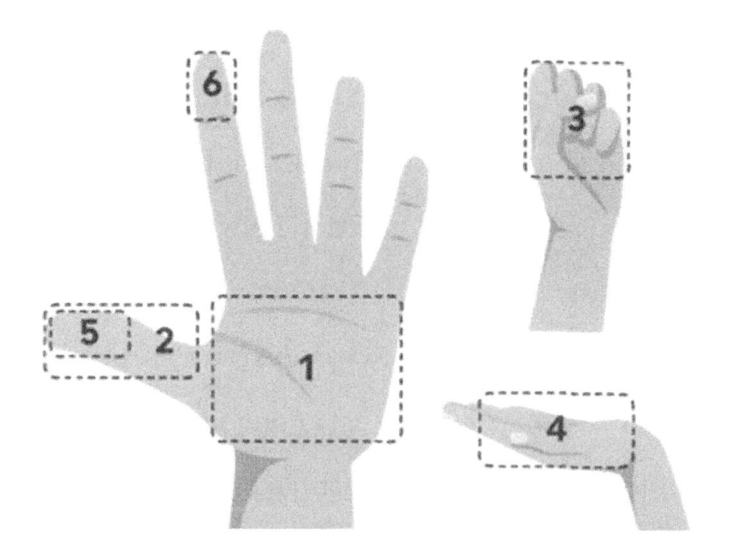

1. 3 ounces of meat, fish, or poultry Palm of hand (no fingers)
2. 1 ounce of meat or cheese Thumb (tip to base)
3. 1 cup or 1 medium fruit Fist
4. 1–2 ounces of nuts or pretzels Cupped hand

5. 1 tablespoon Thumb tip (tip to 1st joint)

6. 1 teaspoon Fingertip (tip to 1st joint)

Calories

Calories are a type of energy that your body consumes and uses to perform physical activities. Do you want to know how many calories you require? Consult an RD/RDN (licensed dietitian or nutritionist).

carbohydrate total

On the label, total carbohydrate refers to all three forms of carbohydrate: sugar, starch, and fiber. When calculating carbs or deciding which items to eat, it's critical to use total grams. A breakdown of the types of carbohydrates in the diet can be found below the Total Carbohydrate (carbs).

Added Sugar

Sugar is one of the three forms of carbohydrates found in food. Labels must contain added sugar as of January 2021 to assist you in distinguishing between sugar that occurs naturally in the item (such as yogurt or fruit) and sugar that was added during processing (like in cookies, candy, and soda). A lot of labels have already made the switch.

Sugar alcohols

Sugar alcohols are sugar substitutes with fewer calories per gram than sugars and starches. Sugar alcohols include sorbitol, xylitol, and mannitol. Sugar alcohols are stated on the label under Total Carbohydrate if a food includes them. It's vital to remember that foods containing sugar alcohols aren't always low in carbohydrates or calories. And just because a package says "sugar-free" on the outside doesn't mean it's calorie or carbohydrate-free on the inside. Always read the label to see how many grams of total carbohydrate and calories

Sodium

The scientific term for salt is sodium. It has no effect on blood

sugar levels. However, on the other hand, excess sodium in your diet raises your risk of high blood pressure and heart disease. You can taste how salty some foods are, such as pickles or bacon. Salad dressings, lunch meat, canned soups, and other packaged goods, for example, have hidden salt. Reading labels might assist you in locating these hidden sources of salt and comparing sodium levels in various items. 2300 milligrams (mg) or less per day is the standard suggestion, whether you have diabetes or not. If you have high blood pressure, talk to your doctor about the best treatment plan for you.

Fats

Total fat is the amount of fat in a single serving of food. In general, to lower your risk of heart disease, replace foods high in saturated fat or trans-fat with foods high in monounsaturated and polyunsaturated fats.

Fiber

Fiber is the portion of plant meals that is not digested or is only partially digested in some cases. Fiber can be found in dried beans like kidney or pinto beans, fruits, vegetables, and entire grains. Your fiber requirements are determined by your age and gender. On average, healthy persons require 25 to 38 grams of fiber per day.

Ingredients' list

Ingredient lists can be extremely useful. The ingredients are listed in order of weight, with the first component accounting for the most weight in the dish. Knowing the contents can help you make healthier choices, such as increasing fiber (look for phrases like whole grain, whole wheat, and so on) or lowering sugar (look for words like cane sugar, agave, maple syrup, honey, etc.).

Percent Daily Values (%DV)

In the right column of the label, you'll find the Percent Daily Values for each nutrient. These percentages show how much of each nutrient the dish delivers if you ate 2,000 calories per day. As a rule, for nutrients like sodium and saturated fat that you wish to limit, aim for fewer than 5%. For minerals like fiber, vitamin D, calcium, and iron, aim for a 20 percent or higher intake.

You won't find nutritional information on everything you buy, but that doesn't mean the remainder of the package isn't full of hints to help you make a better decision. It's crucial to verify the contents list or the back of the pack label before comparing two products per 100g.

Claims on food labels

Many statements on food packaging, such as fat-free or low fat, might be perplexing. Here's the distinction:

You've probably come across the term "net carbohydrates" on food labels. Many food manufacturers make promises about the carbohydrate content of their goods. The FDA does not have a legal definition for "net carbohydrates," and the American Diabetes Association does not utilize them. Always check the Nutrition Facts label for Total Carbohydrate first. You can figure out how specific carbs affect you by checking your blood sugar.

The term "net carbohydrates" isn't the only questionable nutrition claim on food labels. Have you ever wondered what the distinctions are between fat-free, saturated-fat-free, low-fat, reduced-fat, and less-fat foods? The government has defined some claims that can be made on food packaging, and this is what they imply:

Total, saturated and trans fat

- Fat-free: less than 0.5 grams of fat
- Saturated fat-free: less than 0.5 grams of saturated fat
- Trans fat-free: less than 0.5 grams of trans fat
- Low fat: 3 grams or less of total fat
- Low saturated fat: 1 gram or less of saturated fat
- Reduced fat or less fat: at least 25% less fat than the regular version

Sugar

- Sugar-free: less than 0.5 grams of sugar per serving
- Reduced sugar: at least 25% less sugar per serving than the regular version
- No sugar added or without added sugars: no sugar or sugar-containing ingredient is added during processing.

- Although there is no added sugar, there may be naturally existing sugar in the meal.
- Reduced fat or sugar: the product includes at least 30% less fat or sugar than the standard version. This doesn't always imply that it's good for you, and in certain circumstances, the lite version of something like chips can have the same number of calories and fat as the regular version of another brand.

Cholesterol

- Cholesterol free: less than 2 mg per serving
- Low cholesterol: 20 mg or less
- Reduced cholesterol or less cholesterol: at least 25% less cholesterol than the regular version

Calories

- Calories free: less than 5 calories per serving
- Low calorie: 40 calories or less per serving

Fiber

- High fiber: 5 grams or more of fiber per serving
- Good source of fiber: 2.5 to 4.9 grams of fiber per serving

Six ways to be label savvy

- Follow these tips to become an expert at understanding labels in minutes:
- When it comes to traffic light designations, choose for green, amber on rare occasions, and red only as a last resort.
- Percentages of reference intake (RI) are presented per portion and reflect how much the portion contributes to an average adult's daily calorie, fat, sugar, and salt intake. To prevent consuming more calories, fat, or sugar than you require, check how much of the pack counts as a portion.
- Carbohydrates raise blood glucose levels in all people. The number of carbs is not listed on the front of the package; therefore, check the back for the total

carbohydrate, which includes carbohydrates from starchy foods as well as sugars.

- The sugars on traffic lights are total sugars, which does not indicate how much of the sugar originates from natural sources like fructose and how much is added like sucrose or glucose. If syrup, invert syrup, cane sugar, molasses, or anything ending in 'ose' is listed among the first three ingredients, the item probably contains more added sugar. If possible, choose an alternative or limit your portion size.
- On the back of the pack label, look for the fiber content.
- If you're picking between two identical goods and one has more fiber, go for the one with more fiber, as we should all be getting more fiber in our diets.
- Look up the definition of portion size on the manufacturer's website. It could be different from yours and smaller than you'd want! However, if you're trying to lose weight or keep healthy body weight.

Tips for healthy eating for diabetics

1. Consume more fruits and vegetables.

We all know that eating fruits and vegetables is beneficial to our health. It's always a good idea to eat more at mealtimes and snack on them when you're hungry. This can assist you in getting the vitamins, minerals, and fiber your body requires daily to keep you healthy. You might be wondering if you should avoid fruit because it's high in sugar. No, that is not the case. Everyone benefits from whole fruit, and diabetics are no exception. Fruits do contain sugar, but it's sugar that

comes from nature, and this is distinct from the added sugar (also known as free sugars) found in foods such as chocolate, cookies, and cakes. Fruit juices, for example, have additional sugar, so choose whole fruit instead. Fresh, frozen, dry, or tinned fruits and vegetables are all acceptable options (in juice, not in syrup). It's also best to eat it in small portions throughout the day rather than all at once.

2. Choose healthier fats

Fat is essential in our diet since it provides us with energy. However, different forms of fat have distinct effects on our health. Unsalted nuts, seeds, avocados, oily salmon, olive oil, rapeseed oil, and sunflower oil all include healthier fats. Some saturated fats can raise your blood cholesterol levels, increasing your risk of heart disease. These can be found in a variety of animal products and prepared foods, including cookies, cakes, pies, and pastries made with red and processed meat, ghee, butter, and lard. It's still a good idea to use less oil in general, so try grilling, steaming, or baking instead.

3. Reduce the amount of sugar you consume.

We understand that eliminating sugar might be difficult at first, so simple practical swaps are a smart place to start when attempting to reduce sugar consumption. Sugary drinks, energy drinks, and fruit juices can all be replaced with water, plain milk, or sugar-free tea and coffee. To assist you in lowering calories, low-calorie or zero-calorie sweeteners (also known as artificial sweeteners) can be used. Eliminating these additional sugars will help you maintain a healthy weight and control your blood glucose levels. If your diabetes treatment causes you to have hypos and you cure them with sugary drinks, this is still vital for your diabetes management and should not be eliminated. However, if you are experiencing frequent hypos, it is critical to speak with your diabetes team.

4. Get your minerals and vitamins from foods

Mineral, and vitamin supplements do not appear to assist you in managing your diabetes. You don't need to take supplements unless your healthcare provider has advised you to, such as folic acid for pregnancy. It's preferable to get your essential nutrients by eating a variety of foods. This is because some supplements can interfere with your prescriptions or exacerbate diabetes problems such as renal damage.

5. Consume alcohol in moderation.

Alcohol is heavy in calories, so consider cutting back on your drinking if you're attempting to lose weight. Try to limit yourself to 14 units per week. Spread it out to avoid binge drinking and go alcohol-free for several days a week. It's also not a good idea to drink on an empty stomach if you use insulin or other diabetes treatments, and this is because alcohol might increase the likelihood of hypos.

6. Choose healthy carbohydrates

Because all carbohydrates affect blood glucose levels, it's critical to understand which foods include carbohydrates. Choose carbohydrate-rich foods that are low in fat and sodium and keep track of your portion amounts. Like brown

rice, buckwheat, and whole oats are examples of whole grains.

Fruits and vegetables, as well as pulses like chickpeas, beans, and lentils, and dairy products such unsweetened yogurt and milk similarly avoid foods poor in fiber, such as white bread, white rice, and highly processed cereals, must be avoided. If you're not sure, look at the labels of foods to see if they're high in fiber.

7. Reduce your intake of red and processed meat.

If you're reducing your carb intake, you may find yourself eating larger servings of meat to keep you satisfied. This is not recommended for red and processed meats such as ham, bacon, sausages, beef, and lamb. All of these have been linked to heart disease and cancer. Substitute these for red and processed meat: beans, lentils, pulses, fish: eggs, and poultry.

Beans, peas, and lentils are also high in fiber and have a low impact on blood glucose levels, making them a good substitute for processed and red meat and keeping you satisfied. Most people are aware that fish is healthy, but oily fish such as salmon and mackerel are even better. These are high in omega-3 fatty acids, which help protect your heart. Try to consume two portions of oily fish per week.

8. Consume less salt.

Salt consumption raises the risk of high blood pressure, which raises the risk of heart disease and stroke. And if you have diabetes, and you're already at a higher risk of developing all these problems. Limit your salt intake to no more than 6g (one teaspoonful) per day. Many pre-packaged goods already include salt, so study the labels and choose the ones with the least amount of salt. Cooking from scratch allows you to keep track of how much salt you consume. To add that extra flavor, you may also be creative and substitute different types of herbs and spices for salt.

9. Snacks should be chosen carefully.

Instead of crisps, chips, cookies, and chocolates, pick yogurts, unsalted almonds, seeds, fruits, and vegetables as a snack. But keep an eye on your portions, and it'll help you stay on track with your weight.

10. Remember to keep moving.

Being more physically active and eating healthy go hand in hand. It can assist you in managing your diabetes while also lowering your risk of heart disease. This is because it helps your body use insulin more efficiently by increasing the amount of glucose utilized by your muscles. Aim for at least 150 minutes of moderate-intensity physical activity every week. Any action that causes your heart rate to increase and your body temperature to rise. You should be able to talk and only slightly out of breath at this point. You don't have to complete all 150 minutes at once. Break it up into 10-minute portions throughout the week, or 30 minutes five times a week.

Meal planning

Meal planning entails more than just deciding what you'll eat. It's all about choosing wise choices that fit your lifestyle and preferences, as well as what's safe for diabetes management. Once you've mastered the fundamentals, you'll be a pro in no time.

It's no easy chore to time meals to keep blood sugar levels in check. Learn how to make your life easier by following these suggestions.

Learn how to eat healthily to protect your heart. It all comes down to choosing the greatest decisions for you in terms of saturated fats, sodium, and portion control. The more you do it, the less difficult it becomes. Learn to be heart smart. It's vital to eat well, but it can be difficult to know what to eat and how much to eat, especially if you have diabetes. If you're searching for a simple way to get started, try the Diabetes Plate Method. This easy-to-follow guide eliminates the stress of portion planning by eliminating the need for counting, calculating, or measuring.

Diabetic Plate Method

To begin, get a 9-inch plate. Half of your plate should be non-starchy veggies, one quarter should be protein meals, and the remaining quarter should be carbohydrate items. Top it off with a glass of water or another zero-calorie drink, and you've got yourself a well-balanced plate. This helps take the guesswork out of meal planning so you can spend more time doing the things you love. It's very easy to eat more than you require without even realizing it. The plate method is a simple, visual way to ensure that you eat enough no starchy vegetables and lean protein while limiting your intake of higher-carb foods that have the greatest impact on your blood sugar.

Non-starch vegetables

There are two types of vegetables which are starchy and non-starchy vegetables. If you have diabetes, you have typically heard that everyone can eat more of non-starchy veggies, which can help you feel full and contain vitamins, minerals, fiber, and phytochemicals with few calories and carbs, everyone can eat more! These vegetables keep you fuller for longer and provide your body with the nutrients it requires while consuming fewer calories and carbs. Broccoli, carrots, cauliflower are examples.

1. Choose sodium-free, fat-free, and sugar-free fresh, frozen, and canned veggies and vegetable juices.
2. Look for canned or frozen vegetables that haven't had any salt added to them on the label.
3. In sauces, frozen or canned veggies have a higher fat and sodium content than fresh vegetables.
4. If you're using canned vegetables containing sodium, drain them and rinse them with water to remove as much sodium as possible.

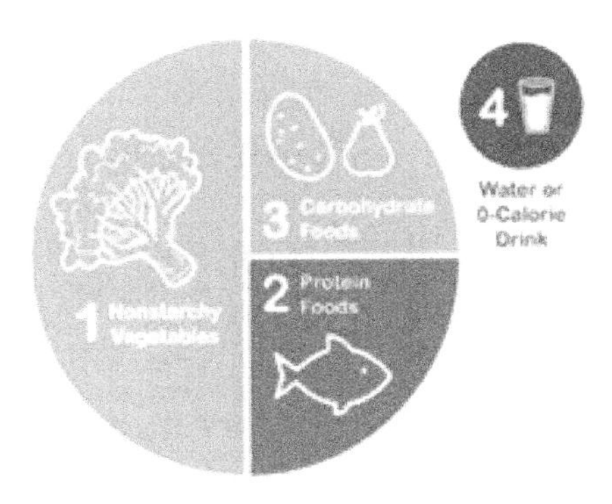

Diabetes superfoods

These are foods that have health benefits, and they are foods rich in vitamins, minerals, and fiber which include.

Beans

Beans including kidney, pinto, navy, and black are high in vitamins and minerals like magnesium and potassium. They're also quite high in fiber. Although beans contain carbohydrates, a 12-cup serving contains the same amount of protein as an ounce of meat without the saturated fat. To save time, use canned beans, but drain and rinse them thoroughly to remove as much salt as possible.

Nuts

An ounce of nuts can provide important healthy fats while also aiding with appetite management. They also contain magnesium and fiber. Omega-3 fatty acids can be found in walnuts and flax seeds, among other nuts and seeds.

Whole grains

It's the whole grain that you're looking for. The word "whole" should be in the first ingredient on the label. Whole grains are high in magnesium, B vitamins, chromium, iron, and folate, among other vitamins and minerals. They're also a good source of fiber. Whole grains include whole oats, quinoa, whole-grain barley, and farro, to name a few.

Yogurt with milk

Milk and yogurt, you may have heard, can help build healthy bones and teeth. Many milk and yogurt products are fortified with vitamin D to make them a rich source of the vitamin. The link between vitamin D and good health is becoming more well-known. Milk and yogurt both include carbohydrates, which should be considered when planning meals if you have diabetes. Look for yogurt that has less fat and sugar added to it.

Omega-3 fatty acid-rich fish

Omega-3 fatty acids may aid in the prevention of heart disease and inflammation. "Fatty fish" refers to fish that are high in these beneficial fats. In this group, salmon is well-known. Herring, sardines, mackerel, trout, and albacore tuna are among the omega-3-rich fish. To avoid the carbs and added calories found in breaded and fried fish, opt for fish that is broiled, roasted, or grilled.

Vegetables with dark green leaves

Dark green leafy vegetables like spinach, collards, and kale are high in vitamins and minerals like vitamin A, C, E, and K, as well as iron, calcium, and potassium. These nutrient-dense foods are also low in calories and carbs, which can be used for salads, soups, and stews.

Berries

Which do you prefer: blueberries, strawberries, or something else? They're all high in antioxidants, vitamins, and fiber, regardless. Berries are an excellent way to fulfill your sweet appetite while also providing vitamin C, vitamin K, manganese, potassium, and fiber.

Tomatoes

The good news is that you're getting critical nutrients like vitamin C, vitamin E, and potassium whether you eat your tomatoes pureed, raw, or in a sauce.

Benefits of meal planning

- It helps you save money because you won't be tempted to get takeout if you know what you're having ahead of time.
- It cuts down on food waste since you'll only buy what you need for the week, and you'll be less inclined to toss out food that's over its expiration date.

- Meal planning saves time because you won't have to make repeated visits to the shop and won't have to think about dinner every night.
- You'll be less stressed if you're organized - meal planning is beneficial for anyone, but it's especially beneficial for people who have busy lives.

Examples of meal plans for diabetic patients

Low -carb diet plan

Eating a low-carb diet means cutting down on the number of carbohydrates (carbs) that consume less than 130g a day. But low-carb eating shouldn't be no-carb eating. Low-carb diets come in a variety of forms. In general, low-carb eating is defined as consuming less than 130 grams of carbohydrates per day.

To put this in perspective, a medium-sized slice of bread contains roughly 15 to 20 grams of carbohydrates, which is about the same as an apple. On the other hand, a large jacket potato can contain up to 90g of carbs, as can one liter of orange juice.

It's not for everyone to follow a low-carb diet. The goal of a low-carb meal plan is to help you maintain a healthy balance while lowering your carb intake. It's nutritionally balanced, with limited calories, and at five servings of fruit and vegetables per day with fiber and protein to assist you in making sure you're

reaching your nutritional needs. Evidence suggests that losing 15 kilograms in three to five months gives persons with type 2 diabetes the best chance of remission. Finding a way to lose weight can also improve your diabetes management and lower your risk of complications. A low-carb diet, for example, is one technique to reduce weight, but there is no one-size-fits-all solution. Weight loss is one of the key advantages of a low-carb diet. This helps persons with type 2 diabetes lower their HbA1c and blood fats like triglycerides and cholesterol; even if you don't have diabetes, a low-carb diet can lower your chance of acquiring type 2 diabetes(Eating Well I ADA, n.d.).

They can be safe and helpful in the short term in helping people with type 2 diabetes manage their weight, blood glucose (sugar) levels, and risk of heart disease, according to the evidence; however, data suggests that they can influence children's growth and so should not be prescribed for children. Furthermore, there is little evidence that this type of diet is beneficial to those with type 1 diabetes. If you decide to adopt a low-carb diet, you should be aware of all the potential benefits as well as how to minimize any hazards.

Following a low-carb diet may raise your risk of hypos if you have diabetes and take insulin or any other diabetic medication that puts you at risk of hypos. Talk to your doctor about it so they can help you change your medications to lower your risk of hypo. Your team may also support you to check your blood sugar levels more often.

Mediterranean diet

High blood pressure and cholesterol, both of which are risk factors for heart disease, have been linked to Mediterranean diets. A Mediterranean-style diet may thus be an excellent choice for people with diabetes, as it helps to reduce the risk of certain diabetes complications. There's also evidence that a Mediterranean-style diet can help people with type 2 diabetes lose weight and manage their blood sugar levels.

This is a plant-based diet that contains a lot of fruits and vegetables, beans and pulses, nuts and seeds, whole grains, and olive oil, among other things. In moderation, it also includes dairy (milk and yogurt), as well as lean protein sources such as chicken, eggs, and fish. Wine is consumed in moderation, and red meat and processed meals are frequently consumed in much lesser amounts.

Vegan diet

Vegan diets are rapidly gaining popularity. A vegan diet is plant-based, which means you don't consume any animal products like dairy, meat, or honey. Most of the vegan cookery is made up of grains, seeds, beans, pulses, nuts, vegetables, and fruits. A well-planned vegan diet can provide all the nutrients you require; certain vitamins and minerals are more difficult to come by in vegan meals. As a result, you might want to take a vegan-friendly vitamin and mineral supplement that includes B12, iodine, vitamin D, and selenium. You could talk to your doctor about it to make sure you're getting the proper dosage. With a vegan diet, one should

- To substitute any dairy products with unsweetened soya milk fortified with calcium, vitamin B12 and iodine.
- It's also crucial to remember to drink enough of water, such as simple water, plain soya milk, and sugar-free tea or coffee.

Conclusion

To conclude, diabetes isn't a death sentence but rather a chronic disease that can be well-managed for healthy living; following all the dietary requirements with 15-30minute physical activities will improve your health status and reduce your risk of diabetes complications. This book provides a lot of information on the nutritional management of diabetes will give other sources to find information from.

Complete this book and have a long life with controlled blood glucose levels without any complications.

References

Boles, A., Kandimalla, R., & Reddy, P. H. (2017). Dynamics of diabetes and obesity: Epidemiological perspective. Biochimica et Biophysica Acta. Molecular Basis of Disease, 1863(5), 1026– 1036. https://doi.org/10.1016/j.bbadis.2017.01.016

Diabetes, D. O. F. (2010). Diagnosis and classification of diabetes mellitus. Diabetes Care, 33(SUPPL. 1). https://doi. org/10.2337/dc10-S062 Eating Well | ADA. (n.d.). Retrieved December 15, 2021, from https://www.diabetes.org/healthy-living/recipes-nutrition/ eating-well Franz, M. J., Boucher, J. L., & Evert, A. B. (2014). Evidence-based diabetes nutrition therapy recommendations are effective: the key is individualization. Diabetes, Metabolic Syndrome and Obesity : Targets and Therapy, 7, 65–72. https://doi.org/10.2147/ DMSO.S45140 Karvonen, M., Tuomilehto, J., Libman, I., & LaPorte, R. (1993). A review of the recent epidemiological data on the worldwide incidence of type 1 (insulin-dependent) diabetes mellitus. World Health Organization DIAMOND Project Group. Diabetologia, 36(10), 883–892. https://doi.org/10.1007/BF02374468

Mignone, L. E., Wu, T., Horowitz, M., & Rayner, C. K. (2015). Whey protein: The "whey" forward for treatment of type 2 diabetes? World Journal of Diabetes, 6(14), 1274–1284. https:// doi.org/10.4239/wjd.v6.i14.1274

Prevention, C. for D. C. and. (2020). National diabetes statistics report, 2020. Atlanta, GA: Centers for Disease Control and Prevention, US Department of Health and Human Services, 12–15.

Sonestedt, E., Lyssenko, V., Ericson, U., Gullberg, B., Wirfält, E., Groop, L., & Orho-Melander, M. (2012). Genetic variation in the glucose-dependent insulinotropic polypeptide receptor modifies the association between carbohydrate and fat intake and risk of type 2 diabetes in the Malmo Diet and Cancer cohort. The Journal of Clinical Endocrinology and Metabolism, 97(5), E810-8.

https://doi.org/10.1210/jc.2011-2444 Stanford, K. I., Middelbeek, R. J. W., & Goodyear, L. J. (2015). Exercise Effects on White Adipose Tissue: Beiging and Metabolic Adaptations. Diabetes, 64(7), 2361–2368. https://doi. org/10.2337/db15-0227

Food Exchange - What is the Food Exchange? (n.d.). Retrieved December 15, 2021, from https://www.diabetes.co.uk/bmi/food-exchange.html

Eating Well | ADA. (n.d.). Retrieved December 15, 2021, from https://www.diabetes.org/healthy-living/recipes-nutrition/ eating-well

Diabetes Complications | ADA. (n.d.). Retrieved December 15, 2021, from https://www.diabetes.org/diabetes/complications

Glycaemic index and diabetes | Diabetes UK. (n.d.). Retrieved December 15, 2021, from https://www.diabetes.org.uk/guide-to-diabetes/enjoy-food/carbohydrates-and-diabetes/glycaemic-index-and-diabetes

Diabetic Exchange Diet - What You Need to Know. (n.d.).

Retrieved December 15, 2021, from https://www.drugs.com/cg/ diabetic-exchange-diet.html

Kandimalla, R., Thirumala, V., & Reddy, P. H. (2017). Is Alzheimer's disease a Type 3 Diabetes? A critical appraisal. BiochimicaetBiophysicaActa.MolecularBasisofDisease,1863(5), 1078–1089. https://doi.org/10.1016/j.bbadis.2016.08.018

Mignone, L. E., Wu, T., Horowitz, M., & Rayner, C. K. (2015). Whey protein: The "whey" forward for treatment of type 2 diabetes? World Journal of Diabetes, 6(14), 1274–1284. https:// doi.org/10.4239/wjd.v6.i14.1274

Karvonen, M., Tuomilehto, J., Libman, I., & LaPorte, R. (1993). A review of the recent epidemiological data on the worldwide incidence of type 1 (insulin-dependent) diabetes mellitus. World Health Organization DIAMOND Project Group. Diabetologia, 36(10), 883–892. https://doi.org/10.1007/BF02374468

Stanford, K. I., Middelbeek, R. J. W., & Goodyear, L. J. (2015). Exercise Effects on White Adipose Tissue: Beiging and

Metabolic Adaptations. Diabetes, 64(7), 2361–2368. https://doi. org/10.2337/db15-0227 de la Monte, S. M., & Wands, J. R. (2008). Alzheimer's disease is type 3 diabetes-evidence reviewed. Journal of Diabetes Science and Technology, 2(6), 1101–1113. https://doi. org/10.1177/193229680800200619

Nelson, R. W., & Lewis, L. D. (1990). Nutritional management of diabetes mellitus. In Seminars in veterinary medicine and surgery (small animal) (Vol. 5, Issue 3).

Boles, A., Kandimalla, R., & Reddy, P. H. (2017). Dynamics of diabetes and obesity: Epidemiological perspective. Biochimica et Biophysica Acta. Molecular Basis of Disease, 1863(5), 1026– 1036. https://doi.org/10.1016/j.bbadis.2017.01.016

Franz, M. J., Boucher, J. L., & Evert, A. B. (2014). Evidence-based diabetes nutrition therapy recommendations are effective:the key is individualization. Diabetes, Metabolic Syndrome and Obesity : Targets and Therapy, 7, 65–72. https://doi.org/10.2147/ DMSO.S45140

Sonestedt, E., Lyssenko, V., Ericson, U., Gullberg, B., Wirfält, E., Groop, L., & Orho-Melander, M. (2012). Genetic variation in the glucose-dependent insulinotropic polypeptide receptor modifies the association between carbohydrate and fat intake and risk of type 2 diabetes in the Malmo Diet and Cancer cohort. The Journal of Clinical Endocrinology and Metabolism, 97(5), E810-8. https://doi.org/10.1210/jc.2011-2444

Wallace, T. C. (2017). MDPI Books. In Batteries (Vol. 2).

Burke, L. E. (1991). Dietary management of hyperlipidemia. Journal of Cardiovascular Nursing, 5(2), 23–33. https://doi. org/10.1097/00005082-199101000-00005

Lal, B. S. (2016). DIABETES : CAUSES, SYMPTOMS, AND TREATMENTS DIABETES : CAUSES, SYMPTOMS, AND TREATMENTS. December.

Alberti, K. G. M. M. (2010). The Classification and Diagnosis of Diabetes Mellitus. In Textbook of Diabetes: Fourth Edition. https://doi.org/10.1002/9781444324808.ch2

Reddy, P. H. (2017). Can Lifestyle Activities control diabetes? Current Research in Diabetes &Obesity Journal, 1(4), 1–9.

http://www.ncbi.nlm.nih.gov/pubmed/29399663%0Ahttp://www.pubmedcentral.nih.gov/ articlerender.fcgi?artid=PMC5792082

Diabetes, D. O. F. (2010). Diagnosis and classification of diabetes mellitus. Diabetes Care, 33(SUPPL. 1). https://doi. org/10.2337/dc10-S062

Astuti, S. I., Arso, S. P., & Wigati, P. A. (2015). 済無No Title No Title No Title. Analisis Standar Pelayanan Minimal Pada Instalasi Rawat Jalan Di RSUD Kota Semarang, 3, 103–111.

Diabetes Meal Planning | CDC. (n.d.). Retrieved December 15, 2021, from https://www.cdc.gov/diabetes/managing/eat-well/meal-plan-method.html

Made in United States
North Haven, CT
31 December 2022